The *Outdoor*
Kama Sutra

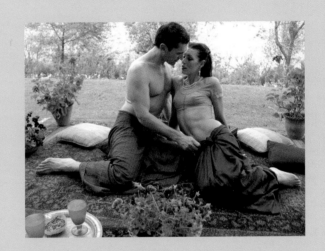

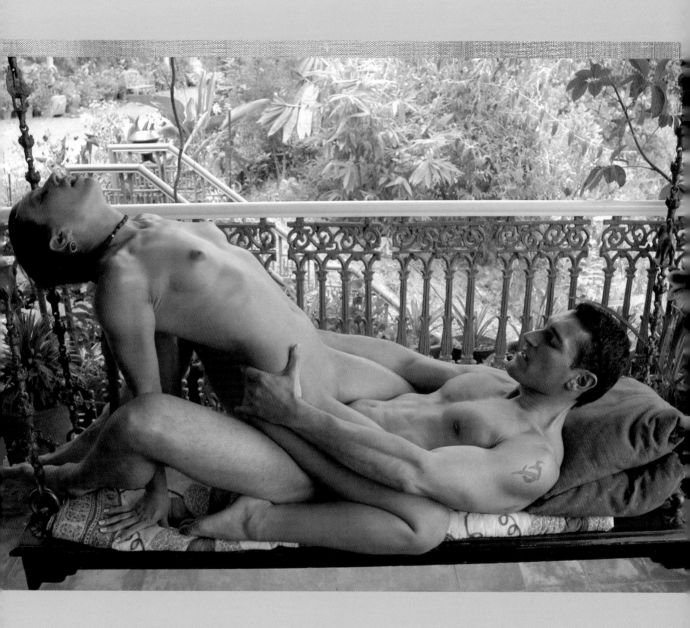

The *Outdoor* *Kama Sutra*

A photographic guide to bringing passionate lovemaking out of the bedroom and into the great outdoors

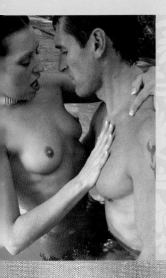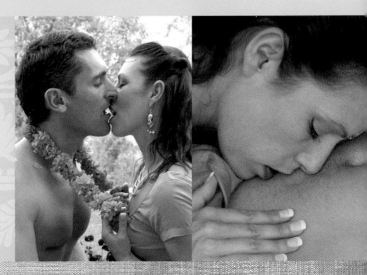

Michelle Pauli

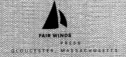

FAIR WINDS
PRESS
GLOUCESTER, MASSACHUSETTS

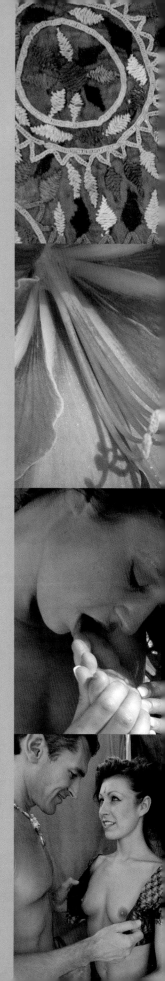

A QUARTO BOOK

10 9 8 7 6 5 4 3 2 1
ISBN 1 59233 179 3

Fair Winds Press
33 Commercial Street
Gloucester, MA 01930
USA

QUAR.OKS
Conceived, designed and produced by
Quarto Publishing plc
The Old Brewery
6 Blundell Street
London N7 9BH

Project Editor Susie May
Designer Alpana Khare
Copy Editor Richard Emerson
Proofreader Claire Waite Brown
Indexer Richard Emerson
Photographer Peter Everard Smith
Assistant Photographer Tai S. Smith
Models Jamie Ross and Natasha Wolek

Art Director Moira Clinch
Publisher Paul Carslake

Photographed in India with the support of
Laburnam Technologies

Color reproduction by PICA Digital,
Singapore
Printed by Star Standard PTE Ltd, Singapore

WARNING
With the prevalence of AIDS and other
sexually transmitted diseases, if you do not
practice safe sex you are risking your life
and your partner's life.

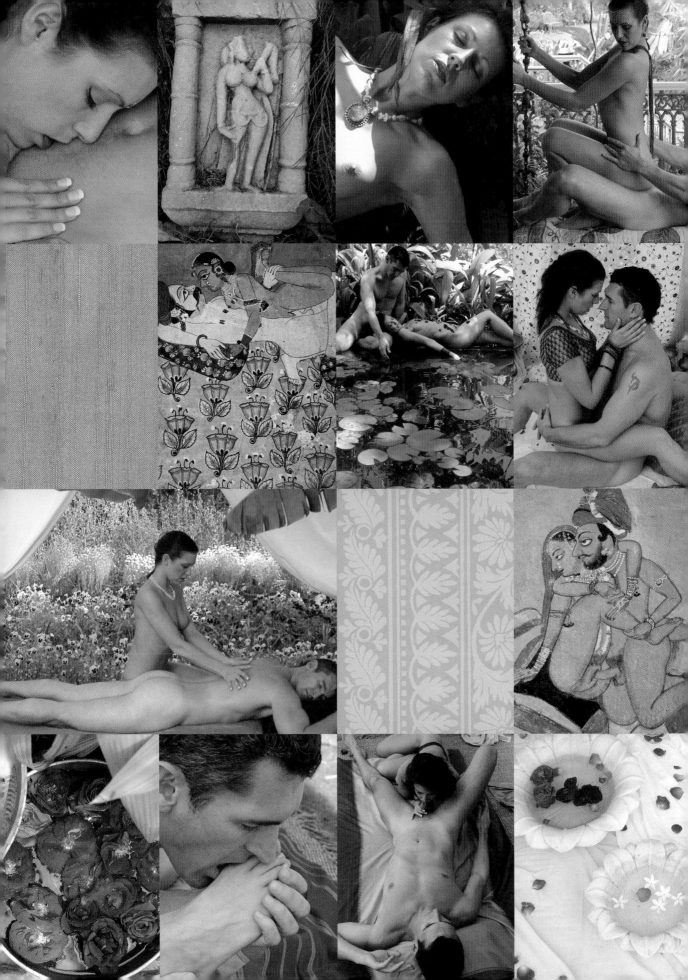

Contents

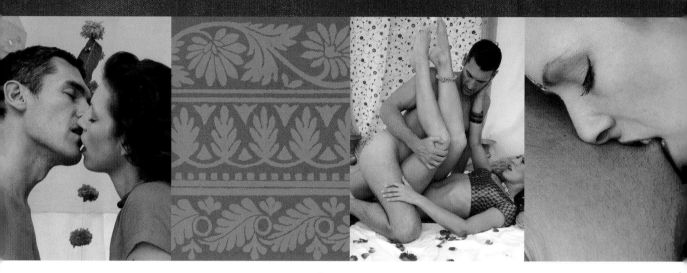

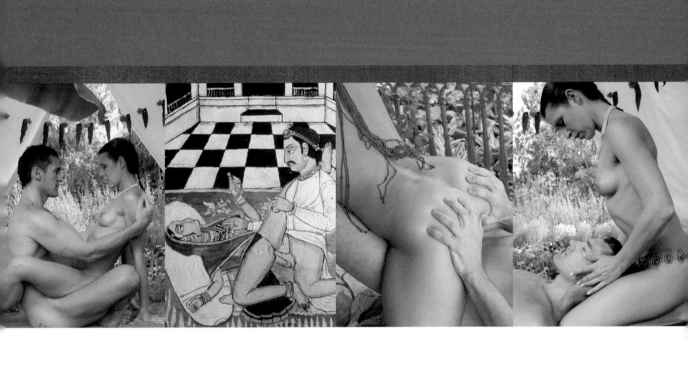

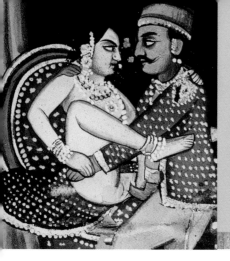

INTRODUCTION:
the Kama Sutra

The Kama Sutra is the all-time classic guide to the art and skills of sex and love. Written between the fourth century B.C.E. and the first century C.E. by a Hindu philosopher, Mallanaga Vatsyayana, the work was not translated into English until the 1880s, and then it was only distributed to a limited circle of enthusiasts, for fear of prosecution.

The Kama Sutra has now become a byword for extraordinary sexual positions, but Vatsyayana's treatise is far more than a simple sex manual. He offers us a thorough exploration of the "science of pleasure" as it was understood in the culture and society of his time for, as he tells us, pleasures are "as necessary for the existence and wellbeing of the body as food."

THE ART OF LOVE

The Kama Sutra offers a holistic approach to the pleasurable life, covering a whole range of man-woman relationships, from courtship and wooing to education and marriage. A disciplined life of enjoyment requires a cultivated body and mind, and Vatsyayana also recommends the intellectual and artistic interests—the 64 arts—that the well-rounded man or woman of his day was expected to know.

BODY, MIND, AND SOUL

"Kama is enjoyment by the five senses of hearing, feeling, seeing, tasting, smelling, assisted by the mind together with the soul."

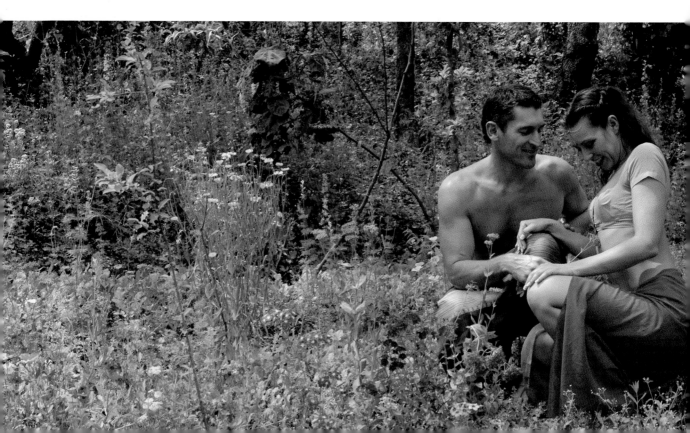

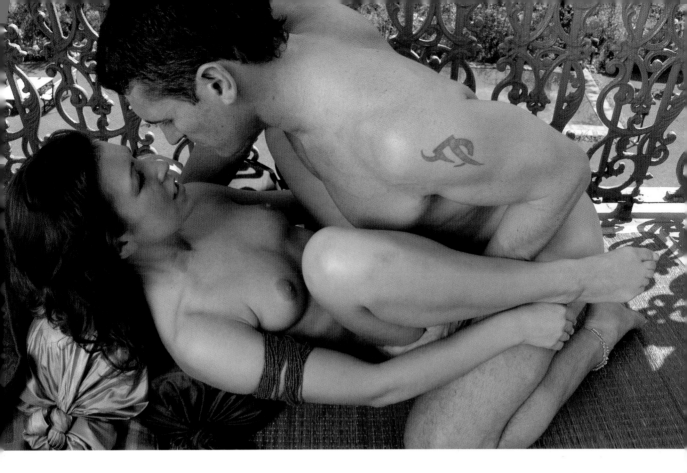

He also teaches that lovemaking encompasses the spirit as well as the body and mind, that it touches something deeper than earthly pleasure, and should be treated as a sacramental and spiritual act.

Of course, not everything Vatsyayana wrote translates appropriately to our society today. Some of it seems sexist and even brutal to our modern-day sensibilities. But the heart of the Kama Sutra, the art of living a life of pleasure and sensuality, and the essential human attributes it explores—love, desire, shyness, intimacy—speak as forcefully to us now, in the West, as it did in fourth-century India. The power and beauty of heartfelt lovemaking transcends all cultures and ages.

THE GREAT OUTDOORS

The Kama Sutra is a celebration of sensuality and the pleasures that flow from it. Nature is the original "sacred space" and making love in the purity of a natural landscape takes us back to our roots, to our own essentially wild, sensual natures. Outdoors you throw off the pressures of your everyday life—the timetables, appointments, clock-watching, day-to-day responsibilities—and gain the freedom to revel in the simple pleasures of the senses: the warmth of the sun on your skin, the scent of pine and wild flowers in the air, the taste of a clear, cold mountain stream.

At its finest, lovemaking in a natural setting is a truly transcendent experience in which you touch something deeper in yourself and in your relationship. You tap into the greater cosmic cycle of the universe—of sex, birth, death, and rebirth—and return to "the source" itself.

Sex in nature is uninhibited and unforgettable. This book celebrates the freedom of wild love and love in the wild.

KAMA LOVE

"Sexual intercourse being a thing dependent on man and woman requires the application of proper means by them, and those means are to be learnt from the Kama Shastra."

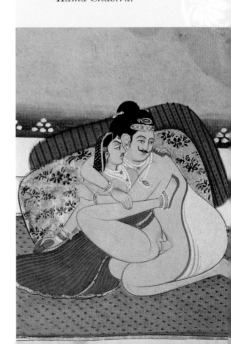

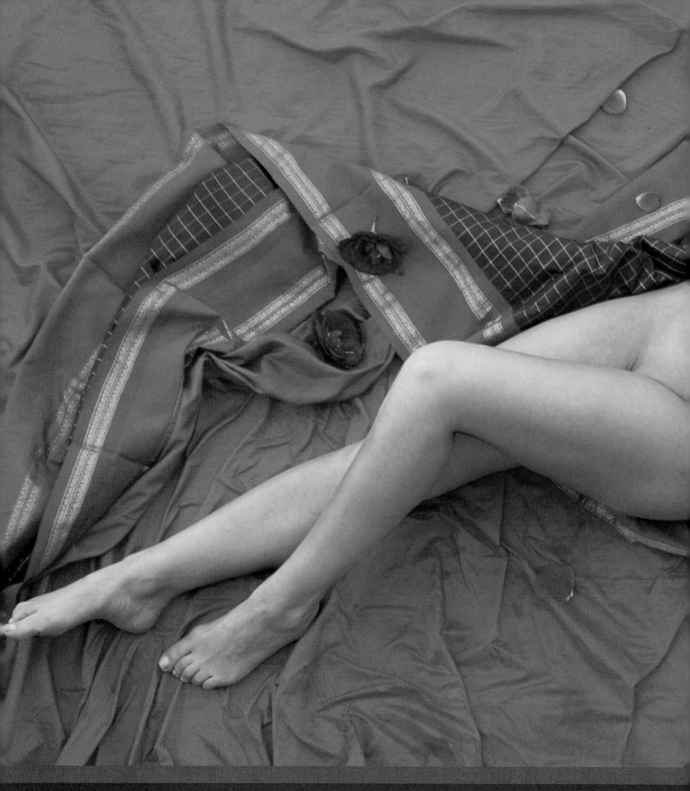

the great

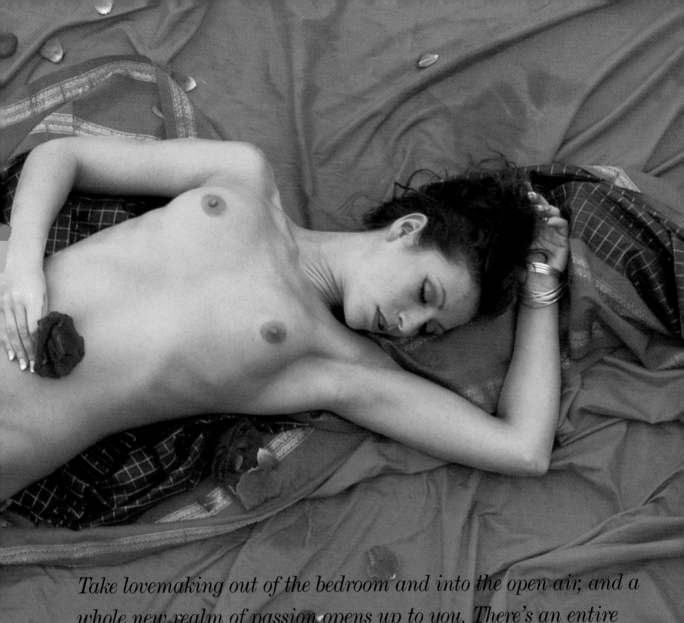

Take lovemaking out of the bedroom and into the open air, and a whole new realm of passion opens up to you. There's an entire wilderness out there to be discovered and a wild side within you waiting to be explored. Making love in nature takes us back to the very roots of our own sensuality and it turns love in the great outdoors into an unforgettable experience.

outdoors

finding wild locations

Outdoor loving can be as close to home as your own backyard or as exotic as making love under a waterfall in the forest. It can involve days of pleasurable anticipation, as you plan your perfect outdoor adventure, or be a totally spontaneous act of passion, when your desire overcomes you in a beautiful natural setting. In this chapter you'll find advice on playing safely in nature, from what to watch out for when searching for the perfect romantic setting to tuning into the cycles of nature. You will also find inspiring suggestions based on the idea of elemental forces, as set out in a traditional spiritual approach of Ayurveda.

ELEMENTAL FORCES

A philosophy and science of healing, Ayurveda has been practiced in India for 3,000 years. At the heart of the system lies five elements—earth, air, water, fire, and space. According to Ayurveda, they are the eternal substances from which all matter in the universe is formed—from a grain of sand to the human body. Each element is a symbol, representing different qualities and characteristics. Understanding the deeper significance of the settings you choose in relation to these elements allows you to look deep into your own essentially wild nature. And the element of space? That's for you to fill in. It is distance and location. In the heart, it is the space that accepts love.

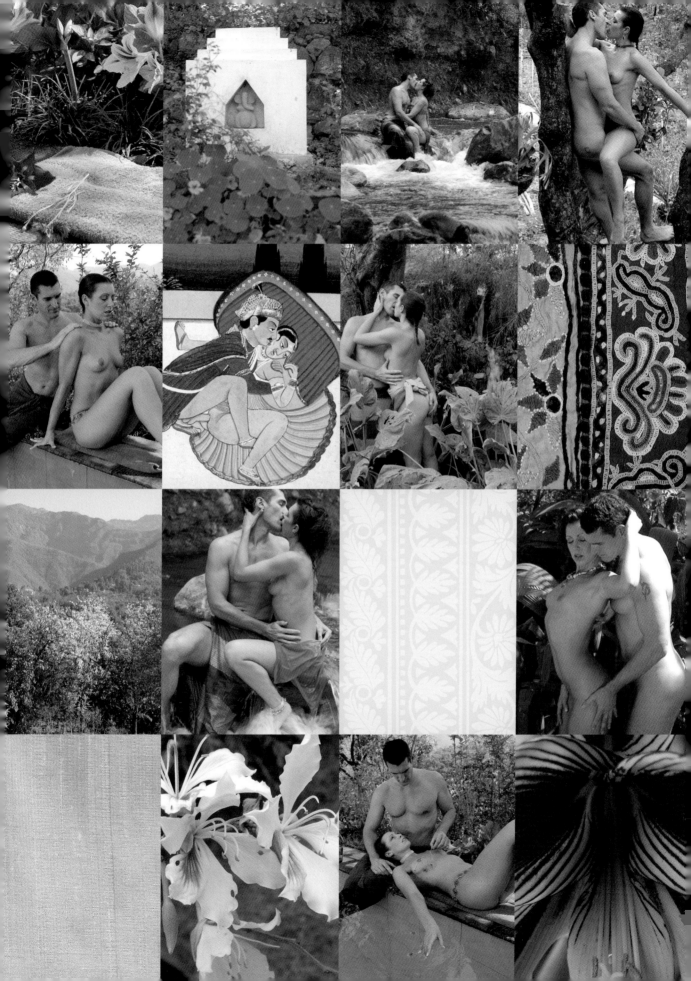

The first step in taking your lovemaking outdoors is to find the ideal setting. Whether you're in an unknown area on holiday or searching out a romantic location closer to home, a little preparation is essential.

choosing your setting

Depending on location, weather, and time of day, the following might be useful:

- Big blanket
- Water
- Bug repellent
- Sunscreen
- Flashlight

There are two approaches to choosing your setting for outdoor sex: the spontaneous and the planned. With the former you're already in the wild and chance upon the ideal location just when your desire is burning. The latter involves more legwork, plus a touch of serendipity, to find that perfect spot you'll want to return to again and again.

Use topographical maps—such as the DeLorme series—to find likely areas, then go off the beaten track. If you find a perfect spot that is occupied, revisit at a different time. Some settings that are busy at weekends and the vacation season could be deserted at other times.

CHECK THE SITE

You've found a "perfect" spot. "Sensible" might be the last emotion you're feeling but, before passion overtakes you, it's worth taking time to check that the location is suitable. First, are you sure it is deserted and you won't be disturbed? This is not just a matter of avoiding embarrassment, there are legal implications (see panel, The Law). Even if there's no one for miles, check for clues that it could be a popular

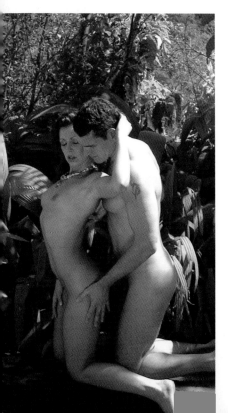

spot—trash cans, well-worn pathways, trespassing notices, and so on.

Dangerous wildlife is another hazard. Are there any signs of animals who might be a problem? If you're on farmland, check for well-maintained fences, indicating livestock are kept within. In the wilderness, make sure you know what to do if you meet with a bear.

The next step is to check for nuisance wildlife. Have you put your blanket down next to an ant hill? Look out for wasps' nests and other bugs that might warrant the use of insect repellent. In deer country, protect bare skin from ticks with sprays containing DEET or permethrin.

Check for problem vegetation such as poison ivy, oak and sumac, bug-filled bark, if you're rolling about in the woods, and dead branches, if playing up in the trees.

TIDY UP

Keep nature natural and aim to have as minimal an impact on the countryside and wildlife you enjoy as possible:

- Before leaving, double-check for paper tissues, clothing, water bottles and other litter, and take it with you.
- Condoms can kill wildlife, so wrap them up and dispose of them at home.
- Don't wash in waterways using soap or oils. Fill a container and wash away from the source.
- Cover your tracks.

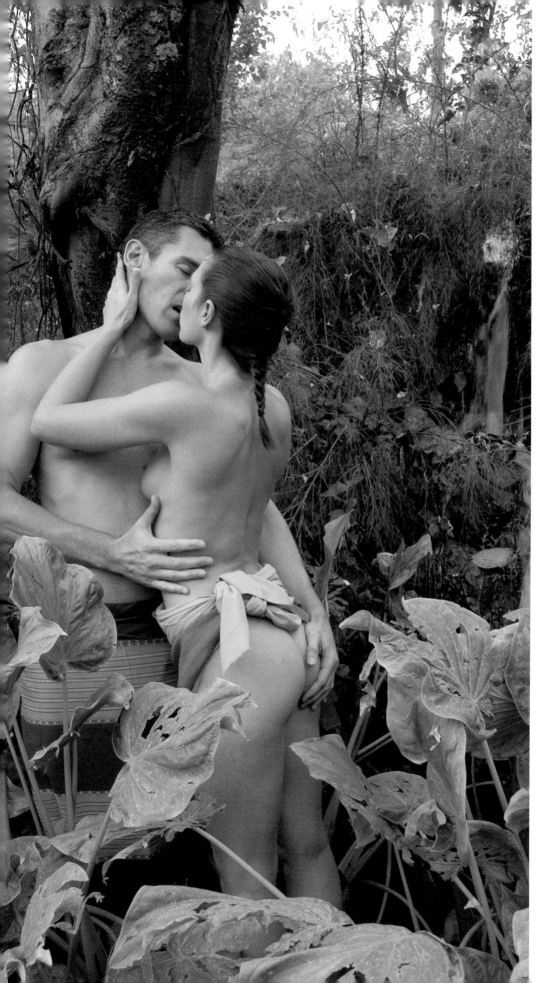

*The perfect wild spot for
love is one you will want
to return to again and
again.*

THE LAW

There are laws to protect
the public from witnessing
sexual behavior or feeling
harassed or intimidated. If
a third party sees your fun
and complains you could
be prosecuted. So choose
your lovemaking location
with care to ensure it is
private and secluded.
Have a cover-up in hand,
such as a big blanket, in
case of an unexpected
visitor. The legal situation
may be different in
individual states.

*Nature's changing mood, as reflected in the weather,
is one of the attractions of outdoor loving—but can
also be one of the pitfalls. A few sensible precautions
will help you avoid getting caught unawares.*

weather wisdom

Feeling the warmth of the sun on your body as you play outdoors is a deeply sexy sensation. Sunburn is less attractive, so enjoy the sun safely. The best form of protection is defense. Don't wait until your skin starts turning pink or feeling uncomfortable before taking action:

- Avoid direct exposure to sunlight between the hours of 11A.M. and 3P.M. when the sun is at its strongest.
- Always use a sunscreen lotion with an S.P.F. (Sun Protection Factor) of at least 15. Use total sunblock on really vulnerable areas, such as nipples.
- Apply sunscreen lotion at least 30 minutes before going out in the sun. Reapply it every couple of hours, as sweat and friction from towels or your lover's body will rub it off.

- Wear waterproof sunscreen lotion when swimming—U.V.A. and U.V.B. rays can penetrate through a yard or so of water. Reapply lotion immediately after swimming, even if using a waterproof type.
- Even with full sun protection, avoid sunstroke by finding shady spots, and keep well hydrated by drinking lots of water.

COLD CONDITIONS

You normally associate passion with heat, but making love in cold conditions is an exhilarating experience too. Nature has a particular beauty in winter and your personal perfect romantic setting may involve cross-country skiing, snow-shoeing, or hiking up a mountain.

Wrap up warmly with layers of clothing, including a hat—most body heat is lost through the head. Take a blanket to cover yourselves and don't forget something waterproof to cover the ground.

SUDDEN WEATHER CHANGES

If you are in an environment where the weather can change suddenly, be prepared. Wear layers of clothing, which you can put on or take off quickly depending on the temperature.

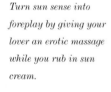

Turn sun sense into foreplay by giving your lover an erotic massage while you rub in sun cream.

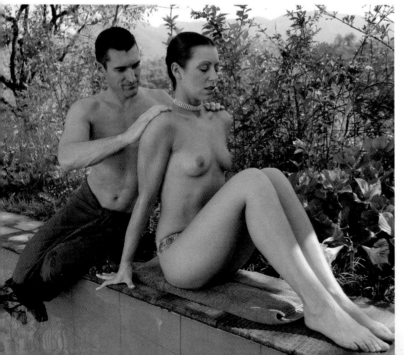

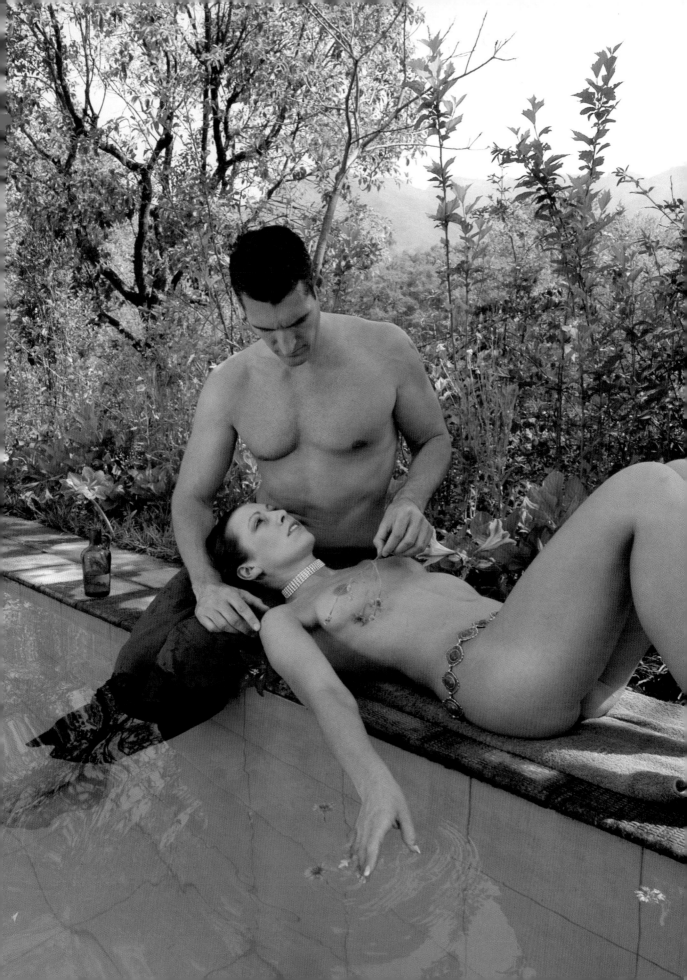

Sensual and wild, "earthy" lovemaking is a celebration of your physical nature, keeping you grounded—literally—and in touch with your primeval passions.

sensual earth

Earth embodies stability, protection, and endurance. As matter in its solid phase, it is a grounding force, providing shape and form. It is *solid* but not *stolid*—the element of earth also represents fertility, sex, and sensuality.

From the briefest contemplation of a patch of earth, its fecundity is clear. It is teeming with life, from insects and worms to the downward thrust of roots and the upward push of shoots. Earth is also associated with ancient wisdom—when you connect with earth you tap into the past, the roots of knowledge.

AN EARTHY SCENARIO

You're playing in the woods, hiding behind trees, having a game of kiss-chase with your lover. The ground feels crunchy with leaves underfoot and twigs snapping as you run about. Breathless, you both come to a stop under an immense ancient oak tree located by

Earthy love puts you in touch with nature's sensuality.

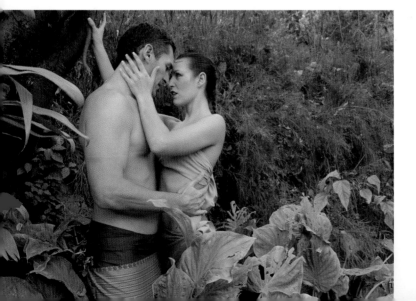

INSPIRATION FOR EARTHY LOCATIONS

Make love almost anywhere in nature and you'll be in touch with earth's sensuality. But some places definitely feel more "earthy" than others—here are some suggestions:
• In the woods
• Among the roots of a tree
• In a huge pile of fallen leaves
• On a mossy bank
• In a cornfield
• In a cave

a mossy bank. Leaning back against the tree trunk, you look up and see a strong branch just within your grasp. You reach out and pull yourself up on to it, urging your lover to follow you up.

Perched facing each other on the branch, nestling in the very heart of the tree, you start to kiss, stroking your lover's skin with one hand and feeling the rough bark of the tree with the other as you grip it tightly.

As your excitement mounts, you climb down—before you both topple off—and roll onto the soft mossy bank. Pulling each other's clothes off, you discover that the love nest you have picked is like green velvet against your skin. With the earthy scent of the woods all around, you make truly wild love.

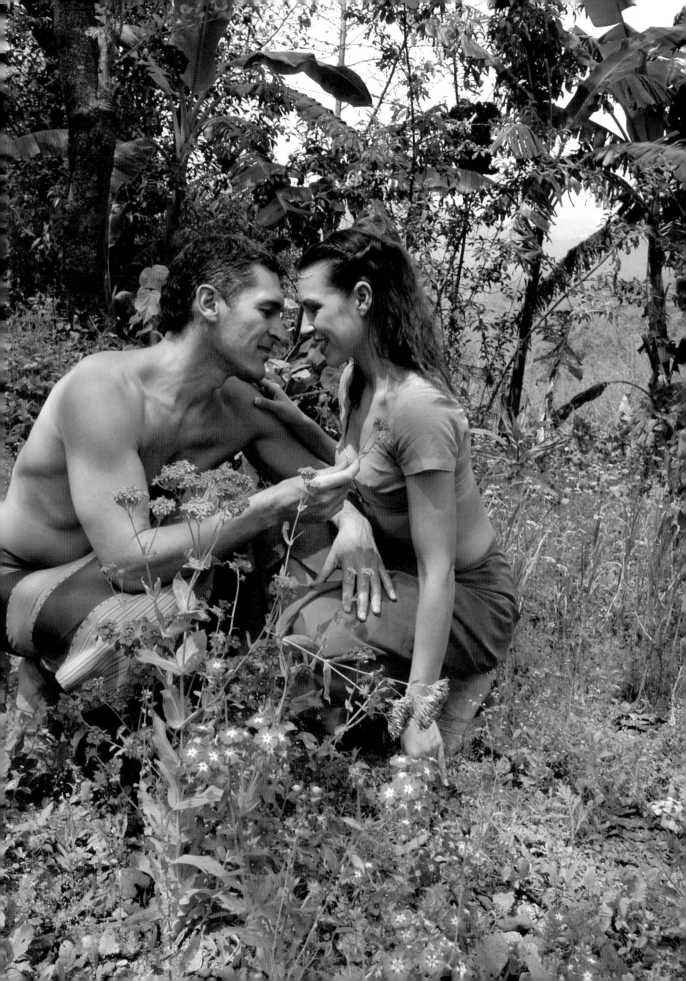

*Quenching your desire for each other on the shores of
a secluded sandy beach, you are completely in flow
with the essential nature of water.*

refreshing water

Pick a watery location and you are going back
to the universal womb, the source of all life. It's
a feminine place, ruled by the rhythms of the
moon and governed by instinct. Water is a
solvent and a lubricant, slowly wearing away
opposition and flowing around tricky
situations; it represents compassion and
tolerance, empathy, and acceptance.

   The element's playfulness is contagious—
make love in water and you'll find yourself
splashing about, ducking under the surface,

*Making love in water is
playful and refreshing—
but be careful!*

INSPIRATION FOR WATERY LOCATIONS
• In the sea
• On the beach
• In a stream
• On the shore of a lake
• On the riverbank
• Under a waterfall
• In an open boat
• On a raft
• In (small) rapids
• In the rainforest

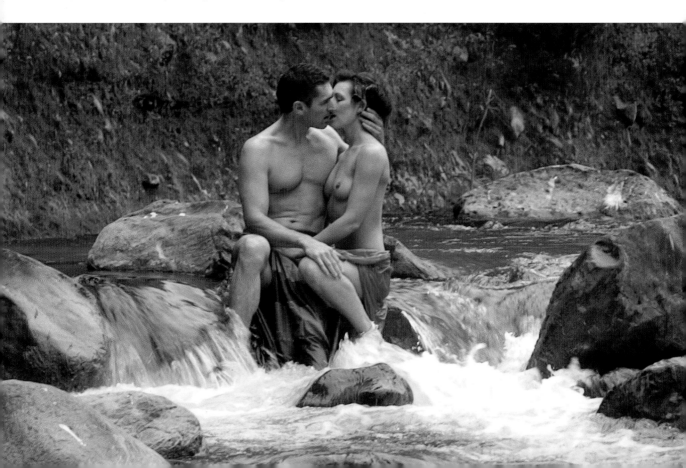

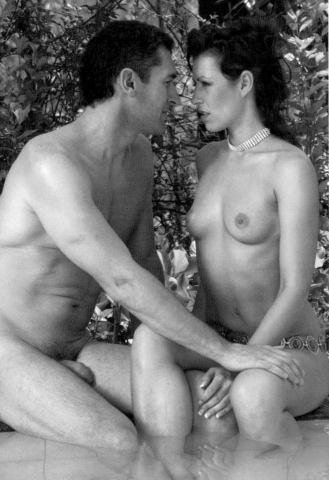

THE ROMANCE OF RAIN

You do not need to be near a watery location to enjoy the element of water if the weather comes to your aid. Making love in a warm summer rainstorm is an incredibly sensual experience. Feel the raindrops on your faces as you kiss. Water falls over your faces and into your mouths as your bodies are refreshed by the water.

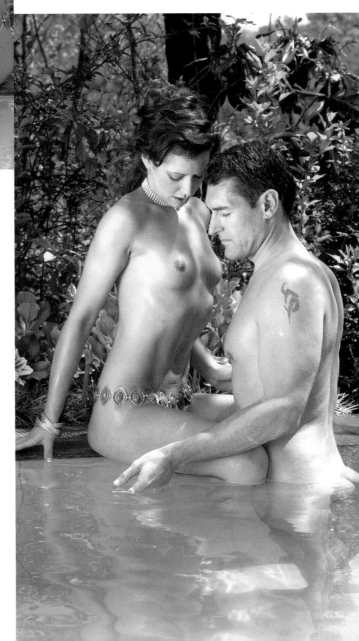

and diving between your lover's legs. You emerge from an encounter with water renewed and refreshed.

A WATERY SCENARIO

Making love on a beach is one of the ultimate sexual fantasies. And one you can put into reality if you find the perfect secluded bay. Perhaps edged by sweet-smelling pine trees, it has soft white sand underfoot and clear, warm water.

You lie naked and enjoy the warm sand between your toes and the feel of your lover's body next to yours. You lean over and kiss passionately, tasting the saltiness on their lips, then slowly massage sunscreen lotion into every part of their body.

Entwining your bodies on the towels you slide against each other, enjoying the heat of the sun's rays. Then, with the heat of passion increasing, you race each other into the warm sea. Embracing, you discover the feeling of weightlessness you get in water, which means making love standing up requires very little effort at all…

Lying entwined with your lover, staring up at a cloudless sky and feeling light of heart and spirit in your love, you are in tune with the spirit of the air.

the freedom of air

INSPIRATION FOR AIRY LOCATIONS

- In the mountains
- In the sand dunes
- In a tree house
- In a hot air balloon
- Underneath a windmill

A gentle breeze or a hurricane, air is the universal breath. It is inspiration—in every sense. Air represents movement and fluidity, the lightness in your heart and step as you walk toward your lover. It is also the sense of space—the feeling that the sky's the limit—as you step out into the unknown with a sense of joy, letting go of all your limitations.

Air governs the winds of change with all the possibilities of freedom and freshness suggested when excitement is in the air. Air is also associated with stillness, light, and intuition. It is the youthful, energetic, humorous side of the element of air that you embrace when the fresh spring breeze tickles the long

grass and you have the urge to take off all your clothes and run about naked through the meadow with your lover.

AN AIRY SCENARIO

It's a beautiful afternoon in the height of summer and you are sitting with your lover on the porch, relaxed after a long lunch and feeling replete with food and love.

Embracing each other, you look out at the clear blue sky, enjoying the warmth of the sun on your bodies and the sound of the cicadas in the meadows beyond. A gentle breeze catches the silk cover on the porch swing and you imagine the sensation of it sliding against

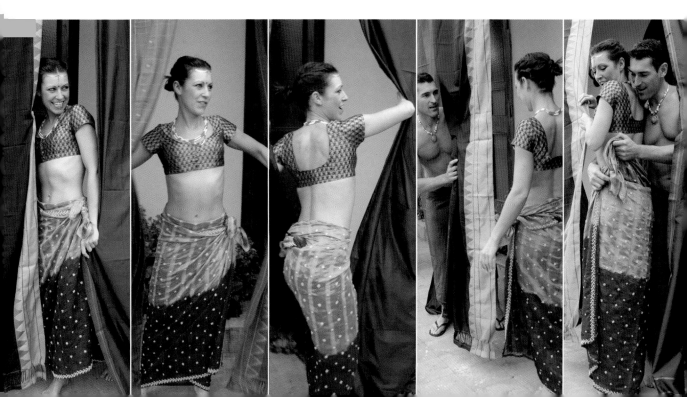

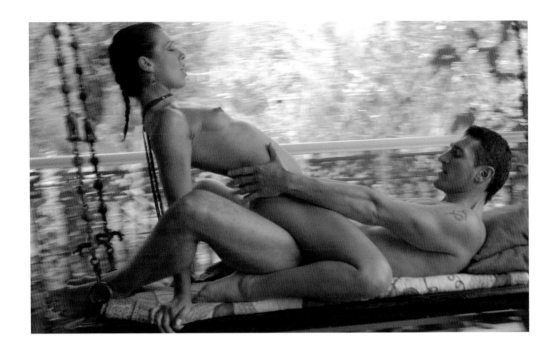

THE ELEMENTS AND THE SENSES

The elements also correspond to our five senses. Sound is transmitted through space/ether, air relates to touch, fire corresponds to sight, water relates to taste, and earth is connected to our sense of smell. When all the senses are used to their fullest and are in balance, then—as in great lovemaking—you are more in tune with the world around you.

your bare skin. You glance mischievously at your lover with a smile, knowing that you are both sharing the same thought and, without a word, you get up and begin to kiss and slowly undress each other. On the swing, the breeze tickles your skin and keeps you cool and the natural movements of the swing through the air provide the perfect rhythm for your love.

A tantilizing game of hide and seek amongst lengths of billowing fabic allows you to discover each other and feel the sensation of the gentle breeze on your skin.

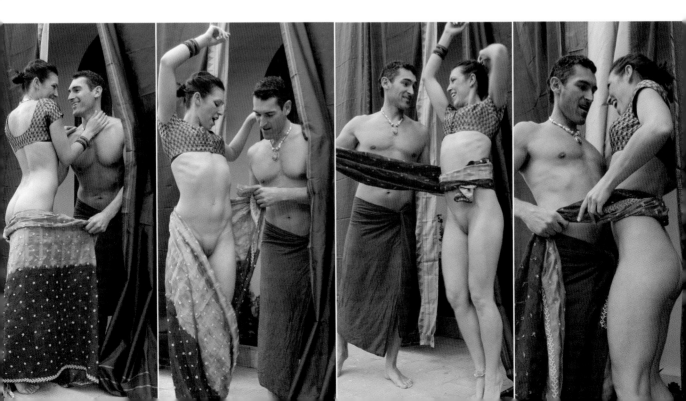

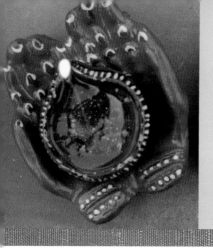

Fire is the element of sexuality, so connect with its red-hot essence by sharing the heat of your passion by a campfire under a starlit sky.

Diwali candles can bring the element of fire to any location.

the passion of fire

Choose a fiery location and you choose excitement and risk-taking. Fire represents burning passion and sizzling sexuality. Through the sun, fire gives us light and heat.
It is a transforming element, turning solids into liquid and then gas—and back again—and converting food into energy.

Fire burns away ignorance, awakening us by removing doubt from the heart and replacing it with joy. Fire is energy, vigor, and flamboyance. It's the fire in your heart that makes you pull your lover toward you spontaneously, and kiss them passionately, wherever you are.

Fire also has its gentle side: think about the delicate flickering flames of the candles you use to make your bedroom a softer, more romantic place for love.

INSPIRATION FOR FIERY LOCATIONS

- By a campfire under a starlit sky
- In a sauna or sweat lodge
- Watching a (distant) firework display
- In the heat of the sun

A FIERY SCENARIO

Take a camping trip into the wilderness with your lover. As night falls, you build and light the campfire and sit by it, faces glowing in the reflected light, a blanket around your shoulders, sharing a glass of warming wine. The sounds of nature at night are all around you: owls hoot and nocturnal wildlife rustles in the undergrowth.

The fire crackles. It's a clear night, so you lie back and gaze up at the stars filling the dark sky. Wrapping the blanket around you both and snuggling closer together, you begin to kiss, cold lips quickly heating up, refreshingly cool hands exploring warm places. Fired-up for love, the blanket slides away and you make love in the flickering light, feeling like primeval man and woman.

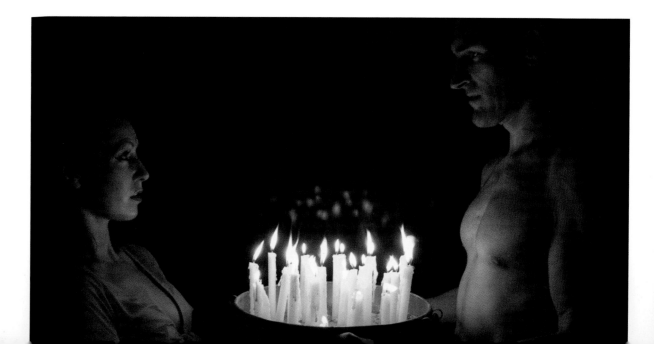

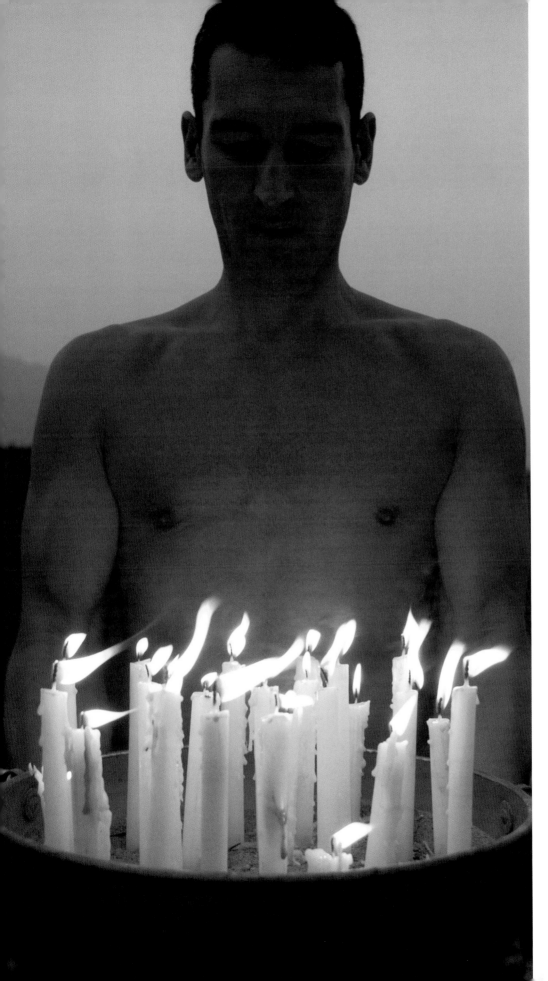

*Finding Wild
Locations*

Candlelight is one of the
simplest ways to turn
any setting into a softer,
more romantic place for
lovemaking.

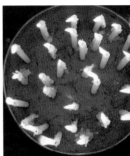

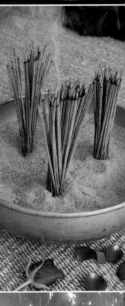

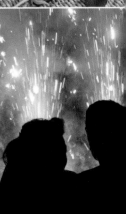

CHAPTER 2
romantic
locations
close to
home

Wild locations are wonderful, but making love outdoors does not have to mean hunting out the most remote hilltop or deserted beach. You can find many exciting possibilities for romantic settings without straying too far from the comforts of home, including backyard hammocks and balcony love nests.

LAWN LUST

For spontaneous passion, everyday locations certainly have their advantages. But with a bit of time for preparation and a dash of imagination you can also take inspiration from the Kama Sutra. Vatsyayana describes in detail the courting man-about-town's beautiful outdoor boudoir of love in which he romances and seduces the object of his desire. So follow his example and create your own sensual garden of delight in a domestic outdoor space.

INDOOR HAVEN

And when weather or time really preclude all outdoor activities, bringing the outdoors in and turning your indoor space into a natural haven continues the spirit of lovemaking in the wild wherever you are.

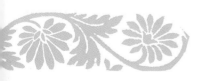

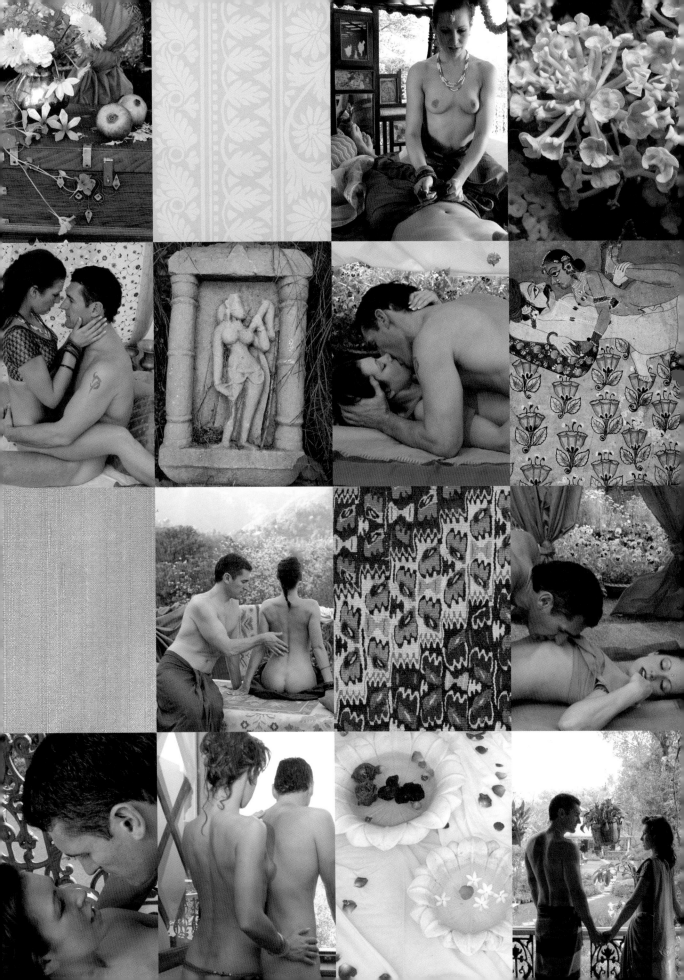

Staying home to make love needn't mean keeping to the bedroom. How about romance under the trees in your own backyard, on a heap of pillows on the patio, or rocking in the porch swing?

everyday locations

When you begin to think about the potential of everyday locations as settings for outdoor romance, you start to see your familiar environment with fresh eyes. As you check out your patio for privacy, test the sturdiness of the porch swing or hammock. Suddenly, places you may not have ever really noticed appear in a whole new light.

Think beyond the bedroom and there is a whole world of possibilities for lovemaking in your own environment.

HOME LOVING

While it may lack the exoticism of the unknown, a familiar location certainly has its advantages: there's no need to travel; all the comforts of home are close by; and the convenience and security is reassuring.

When you have less time to spare, or the weather is cold, you can venture outdoors knowing that you don't have far to go to warm up afterward with a hot drink or bath.

Making love in a rainstorm—a really sensual experience—also holds much more appeal when you know that towels and dry clothes are warming on a radiator a short distance away.

SEXY SURPRISE

But this does not mean that domestic settings lack the element of surprise. It is much easier to prepare a spontaneous romantic treat for your lover when all you need is close to hand.

If the sun comes out during an otherwise lackluster weekend, you can quickly lay out a backyard picnic to share or prepare a candlelit evening picnic on the lawn.

EVERYDAY INSPIRATION

Even the most limited of outdoor spaces can provide opportunities for outside lovemaking in your home environment. A balcony may have space for pillows or even to hang a hammock. A patio or sun deck can be shielded with screens or shrubs. With more space to play in, the options increase: by or in the pool, in the summerhouse, under the trees, in the arbor… Bear in mind, though, that on a still day, sound can travel surprisingly far—you may want to tone down your cries of pleasure accordingly.

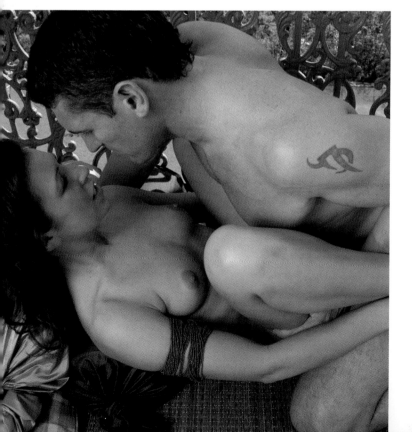

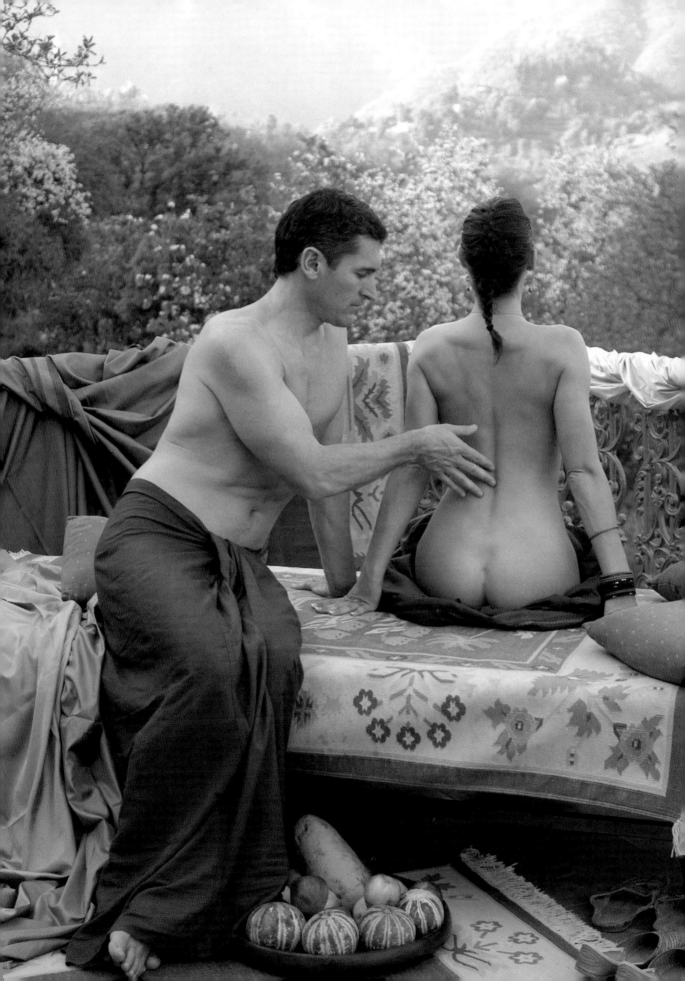

The power of setting aside a special place for love lies not just in the beauty of the surroundings but also in the intention you hold when you create such a space, whatever your setting.

a sacred space

The "ideal citizen" of the Kama Sutra understood the pleasure of having a complete sensual environment for lovemaking. Vatsyayana provides an evocative description of the boudoir of a typical "man-about-town" of the day as a kind of wondrous playroom filled with everything lovers might desire during their time together.

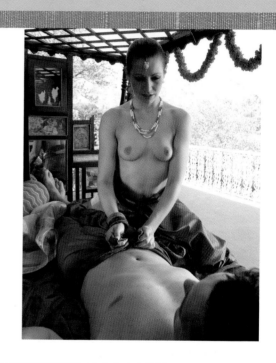

The "outer room," surrounded by the garden, was "balmy with rich perfumes." It featured a soft bed, covered with a clean white cloth and decorated with garlands and bunches of flowers, and with a canopy above. On a nearby stool were placed pots of fragrant

A traditional Kama Sutra boudoir of love would be a sumptuously decorated playroom.

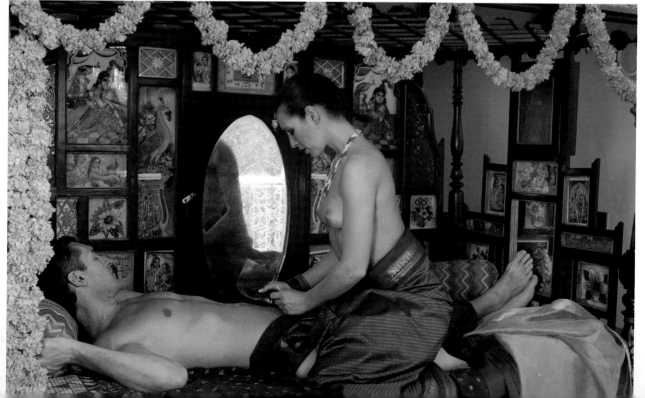

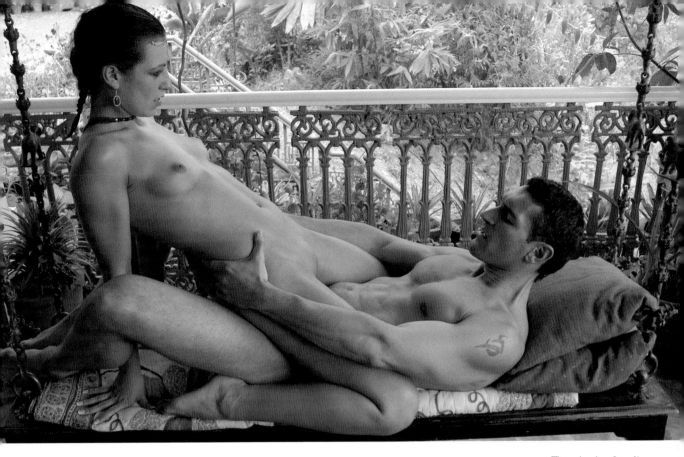

ointments, to be used in the night's pleasures, herbs, and more flowers. There would also be a box of ornaments, books, garlands of yellow amaranth flowers, a drawing board, a lute, and boards for playing games.

GARDEN OF LOVE

In the garden, cages of birds filled the air with their song as the lovers sat under "a bower of creepers covered with flowers." The garden would also feature different types of swings—a favorite prop in Kama Sutra lovemaking. For married couples, the garden was the wife's domain. It would be a place designed to delight the senses, filled with fragrant grasses, herbs, and flowers such as wild jasmine and china rose. It was a place for contemplation and play: "She should also have seats and arbors made in the garden, in the middle of which a well, tank, or pool should be dug."

A SPECIAL PLACE

The notion of a special place for lovemaking is just as relevant today. It is unlikely to be as extravagant as Vatsyayana's description, especially in a spontaneous outdoor setting (although you'll find ideas for creating your

own version in the next few pages). But the basic act of marking out time and space dedicated to lovemaking—even in a simple fashion—helps to set your lovemaking apart as something special.

NATURE'S BOUNTY

In the absence of a Kama Sutra-style boudoir, there are simple ways to do this outdoors, using natural elements. A circle of small rocks is a beautiful and effective way of marking out space. You could also use feathers, twigs, flowers, or a mixture of all the different gifts of nature. The power of the space you make lies in the intention that goes into creating it. As you focus on collecting your objects and setting them out, becoming more present in the moment, it becomes "sacred space" that you and your lover dedicate to each other and your pleasures.

The swing is a favorite prop in the Kama Sutra, and is an exciting place for lovemaking.

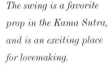

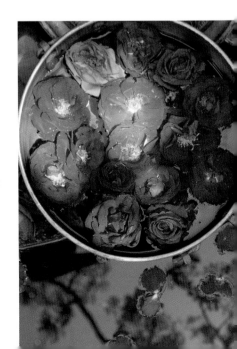

Whatever the size of your outdoor space, with a little care and imagination it is possible to transform it into an outdoor boudoir of love.

creating an outdoor boudoir

For most of us, the Kama Sutra citizen's love nest is a fantasy setting. But whether you have a small garden, a terrace, or a balcony, you can create a romantic environment that captures some of its sensual delights.

LIVING THE FANTASY

The first consideration is seclusion and privacy. It is vital to feel absolutely at ease and comfortable in your space, and that means ensuring that you can't be spied on or embarrass your neighbors. In a large backyard this is less of a problem and you may already have shielding from trees, shrubs, or a summerhouse. In a small, overlooked backyard or a balcony, consider using drapes or screens to create a private place.

Check that lawn furniture is sturdy enough to support you, and that your swing can support your weight. Hammocks are wonderful and full of possibilities. Swimming pools or hot tubs let you incorporate the sensual fun of water into your lovemaking, or a paddling pool can be fun for playful splashing about.

Think about using fast-growing plants, such as passion flower, to create privacy naturally, and soften walls and fences with scented creepers. A classic romantic garden will also feature little hidden corners for trysts, love seats, highly scented flowers, and perhaps an arbor to sit beneath. Encourage wildlife with birdfeeders and a pond.

Drapes, screens, and pot plants are all simple but highly effective ways of creating a private place.

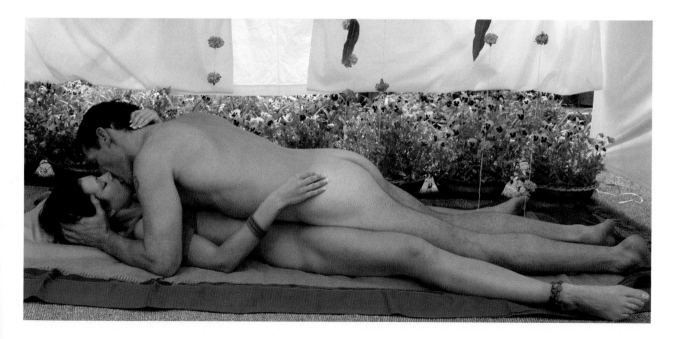

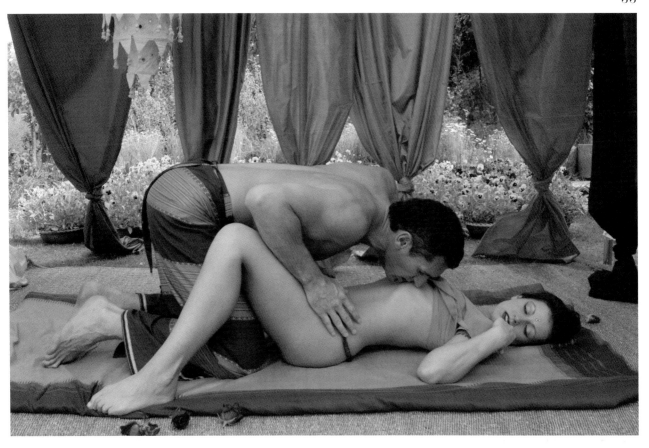

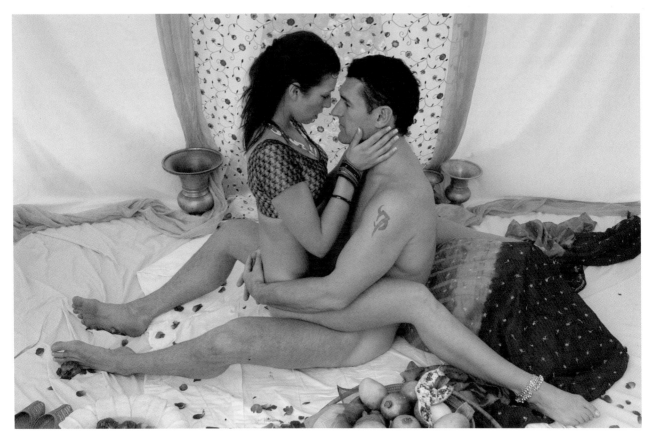

THE GREAT OUTDOORS

Romantic Locations Close to Home

The perfect outdoor boudoir of love will delight all your senses and contain all that you need for an afternoon of pure pleasure.

A FEAST FOR THE SENSES

Your outdoor boudoir should include aspects that delight all the senses.

- Taste: grow juicy fruits, such as strawberries and raspberries. If that's not possible, have a tray of prepared fresh fruit cut into small pieces.
- Touch: use fabrics that feel luscious on bare skin, such as velvet and silk.
- Sight: make the most of the natural surroundings. Place your bed area under a tree so that you can lie back and look into its wonderful canopy of branches.
- Scent: fresh flowers and herbs provide gorgeous natural aromas.
- Sound: to the sounds of nature, such as birdsong, add wind-chimes (choose wooden types for a mellow sound) or small bells that tinkle in the breeze.

Another approach to adding romantic and sensual touches to your outdoor boudoir is to emphasize the natural elements:

- Water: a water feature is beautifully calming to look at and listen to.
- Fire: create a fire pit in a larger setting, or use outdoor candles and lanterns in a smaller one.
- Air: swathes of silk hanging from branches or hooks on a balcony swish in the breeze and can also shield your space.
- Earth: use pots with herbs and plants to represent this element.

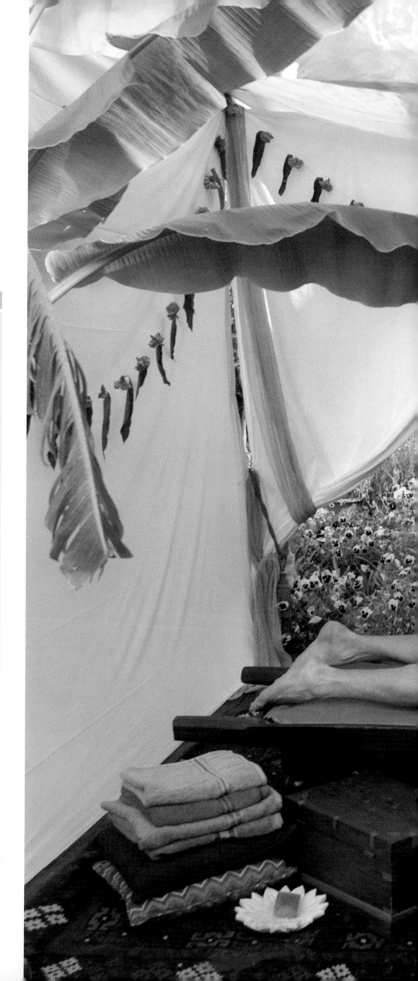

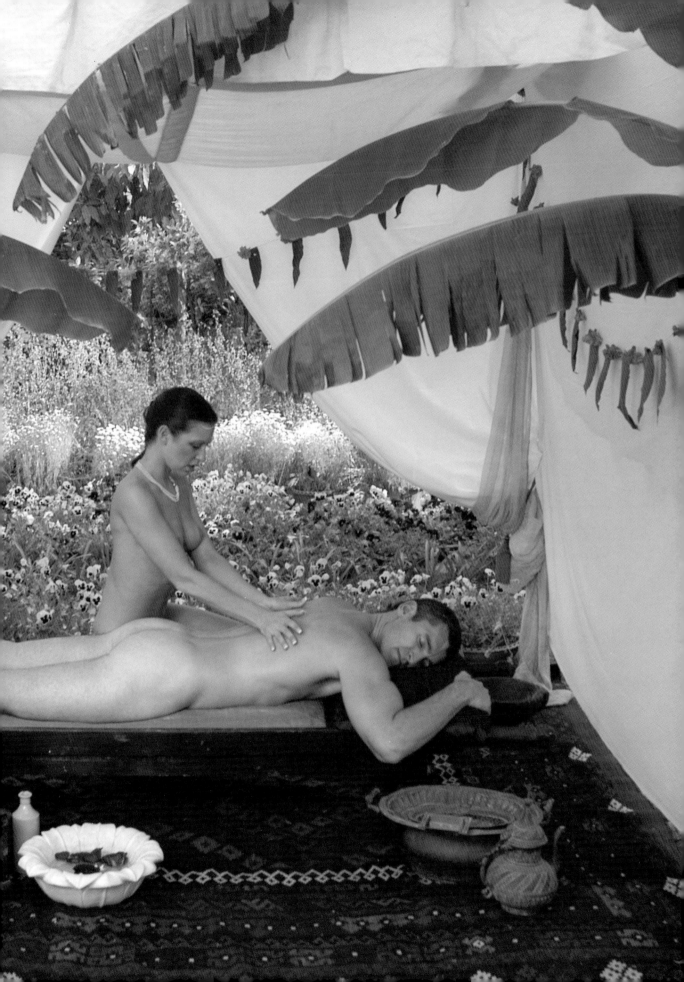

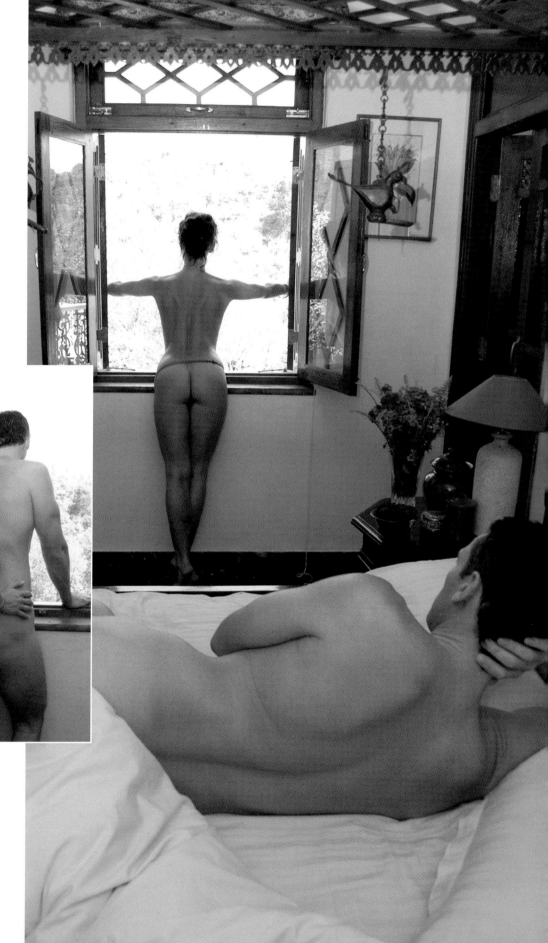

*Bringing the outdoors in
can be as simple as
opening a window to feel
the fresh air on your
bodies.*

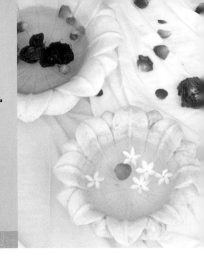

Spending time outdoors with your lover may not always be feasible because of inclement weather or time constraints, but you can bring the outdoors in and give your home the spirit of the wild.

bringing the outdoors in

The principle of making the location for your lovemaking your special sacred space applies indoors as well as out. Perhaps you always make love in the same place, but there are no rules that say that sex has to be reserved for the bedroom. Now is the time to rethink old patterns. Step out of those ingrained habits and apply the freedom of spirit of outdoor lovemaking to inside your home.

Think about whether you can create a temporary romantic space for lovemaking that incorporates some of the elements of love in the wild. For example, place some pillows by an open window so that you can see the sky and feel fresh air on your bodies.

ROMANTIC TOUCHES
Sectioning off an intimate space using drapes and hangings can work well for creating a sense of "space out of time," which takes your minds away from the domestic surroundings. Make up a soft area to lie on with pillows, fake fur rugs, and soft bedding. For an extra romantic touch, you might decide to scatter rose petals on the floor and bedding. You could also create a circle around your bed area with stones, flowers, and bowls of water.

Remove objects such as the television and computer from sight, or cover them with a cloth, and make sure the telephone ringer is switched off and the answering machine is turned down. Keep the lighting as natural as possible and after dark use candles rather than harsh electric lights.

Fresh flowers and plants are a very easy way of bringing the outdoors inside. If the flowers aren't highly scented, then essential oils in a burner provide a much more natural scent than incense. Use shells, feathers, pebbles, driftwood, and other finds from times you have shared outdoors to put you in touch with nature and remind you of your al fresco adventures. Another attractive option is an indoor water feature, or bowls of water with floating candles.

If your indoor space suffers from traffic sounds or noisy neighbors then CDs of natural sounds such as birdsong are ideal for transporting you away from urban life.

A SEASONAL ALTAR

A "seasonal altar" is an evocative reminder of the natural world and its rhythms. Cover a low table, box, or shelf with beautiful fabric and create an arrangement of natural objects: spring bulbs, summer flowers, colorful fall leaves, changing the display with the passing seasons.

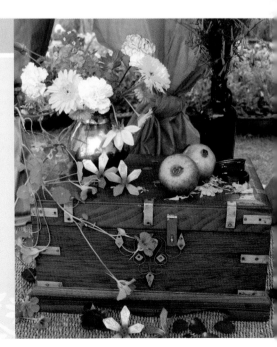

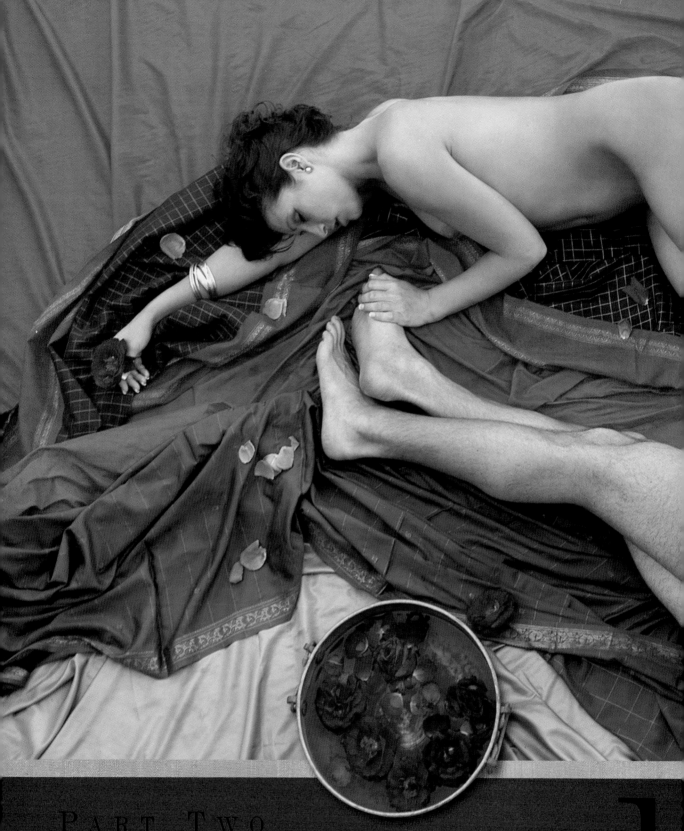

PART TWO

in the mood

Getting in the mood for love is a journey of the mind, body, and spirit, as you awaken every part of your being to the pleasures of sensual love. From wooing your lover to embracing, kissing, and tantalizing touch, prolonging the tension of the sexual build-up is an art in itself.

for love

CHAPTER 3

the sensual body and mind

The greatest pleasures come to those who wait, and the Kama Sutra teaches you simply to slow down. Lovemaking begins long before intercourse takes place. Gently awakening the body and mind to intimate and loving feelings offers a tantalizing promise of what is to come.

SENSUAL AWAKENING

The sensual body is alive to its potential for total pleasure. Celebrating your body—by loving it and exploring it—is the first step on this journey. Awakening the body during foreplay by arousing it with a variety of sensations sets the scene for heightened pleasures during lovemaking. In this chapter, discover a fun and creative way to delight all the senses outdoors with a "sensual picnic basket."

Being in the mood for love is also a journey of the mind. In the time of the Kama Sutra lovers were courted in ways still recognized today—love talk, gifts, and shared leisure activities.

CONNECT WITH YOUR LOVER

On a more subtle level, when you let go of distractions so that you really connect with your lover and can be fully present in the moment you are sharing, you are making the most of your time together. This chapter offers inspiration to help you make that connection.

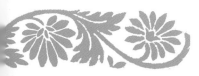

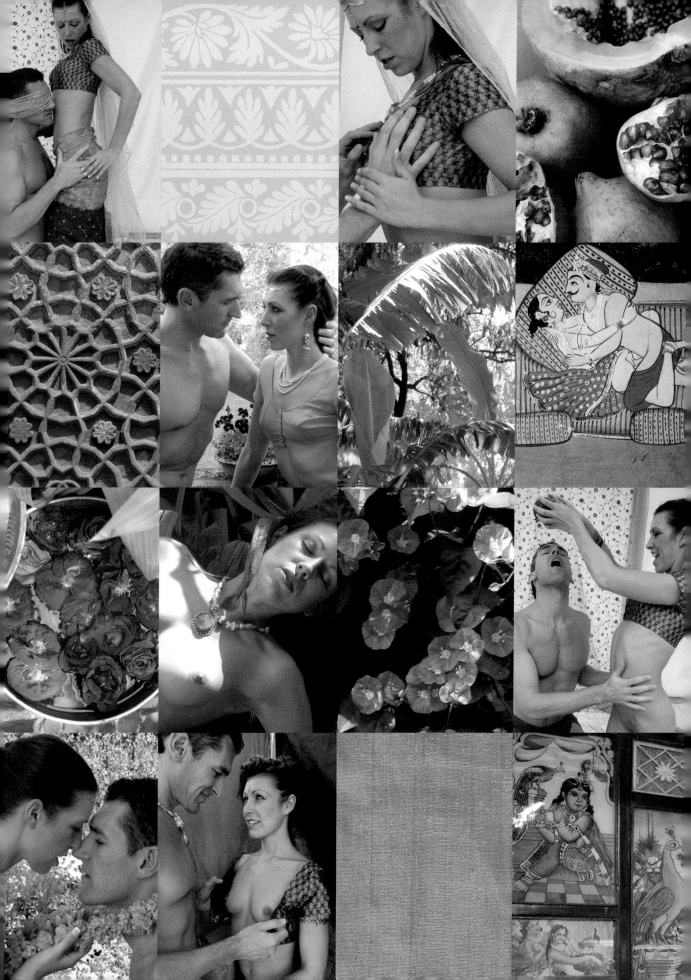

Awakening your body ready for the pleasures of lovemaking is a celebration of the joy of being a sexual being. Treating your body with reverence, loving it and preparing it for lovemaking, is part of that celebration.

the sensual body

One of the joys of making love in nature is that it helps you to shed your everyday, urban concerns and replace them with the recognition that, simply by being, you are part of the natural world.

Feeling at home and comfortable in your body is a cornerstone of relaxed, uninhibited and—most importantly—joyful lovemaking. Many people find it difficult to love their bodies. There is always a part that is too big, too small, too wobbly or, somehow, just not good enough.

The Kama Sutra teaches that your body is a sacred object to be treated with reverence.

ACCEPT YOURSELF

In order to befriend your body you need to acknowledge its "naturalness." Try to see it as part of the natural landscape. As a rule, you don't judge nature with a critical eye, deciding "that mountain really should be smaller" or "that meadow should be flatter." You accept nature as being just right as it is.

Do the same with your body. Look at it with a true lover's non-critical eye and recognize it as being perfect just as it is—part of the great natural order.

The Kama Sutra teaches that the body should be treated as a sacred object and that preparing the body for sex—a sacred act— recognizes that reverence. A householder in Vatsyayana's time would take great care of his body, ensuring that it was ready for the sensual pleasures in store (see panel below).

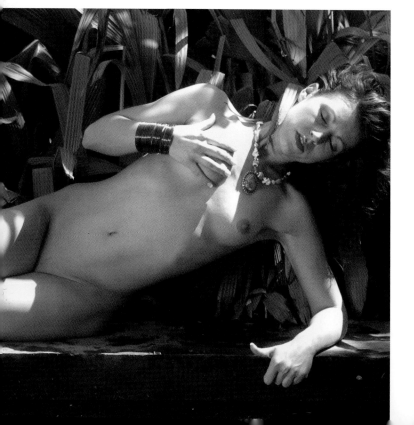

THE MAN'S DUTY

"He should bathe daily, anoint his body with oil every other day, apply a lathering substance to his body every three days, get his head (including face) shaved every four days and the other parts of his body every five or ten days. All these things should be done without fail, and the sweat of the armpits should also be removed."

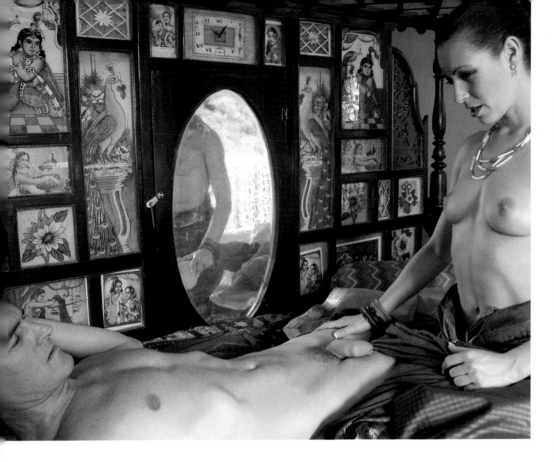

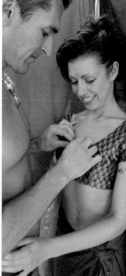

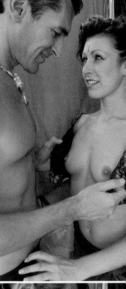

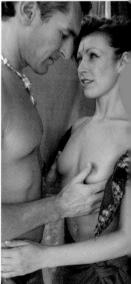

BATHE IN THE ELEMENTS

Cleansing before lovemaking is not just a matter of sexual hygiene, it also marks a change of mental state, washing away the cares of the day. As an alternative to showering with your lover before setting off on your outdoor adventure, you'll find bathing in nature, using natural elements, both refreshing and fun.

Use whatever is around you—stream, lake or sea—to splash in with your lover. If you are in an arid landscape use a bottle of drinking water to bathe your hands and feet.

Bathing can involve all the elements, not just water. If the weather is mild, have an exhilarating "air bath"—take off your clothes and feel the fresh air on your naked skin.

Try a fiery "sun bath." Enjoy the nourishing energy of sunlight all over your naked body for a few moments before covering up or seeking the shade.

A messy and fun option is a mud bath—rub a handful of mud over your body, or let your lover do it for you. Mud also makes a great exfoliant, but ensure there is clean water to hand to wash it off.

Awakening your body for sensual lovemaking begins with recognizing that it is perfect as it is. Wearing small items of clothing such as a cropped blouse or "choli," or loose items such as a sarong, will give you the opportunity to enjoy undressing each other.

THE WOMAN'S DUTY

"When the wife wants to approach her husband in private her dress should consist of many ornaments, various kinds of flowers, and a cloth decorated with different colors, and some sweet-smelling ointments or unguents."

IN THE MOOD
FOR LOVE

*The Sensual
Body and Mind*

*Appreciating all the
elements of nature with
your lover will bring you
to a place of stillness and
serenity in which you
can let go of distractions
and truly connect with
each other.*

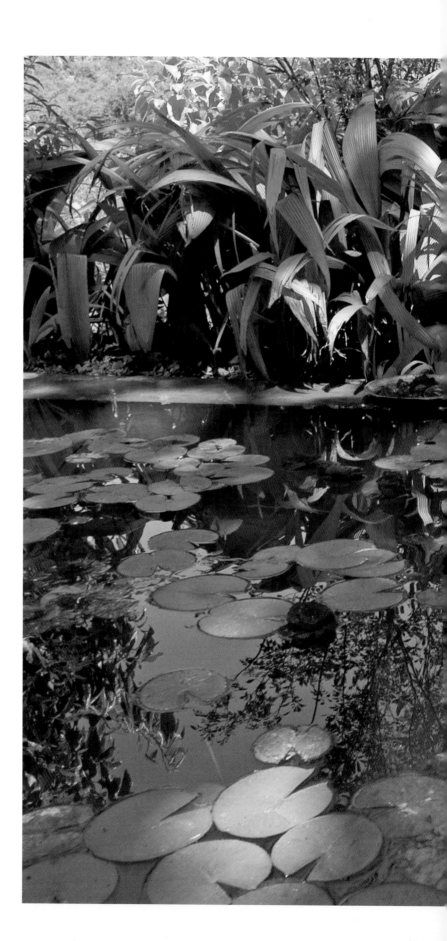

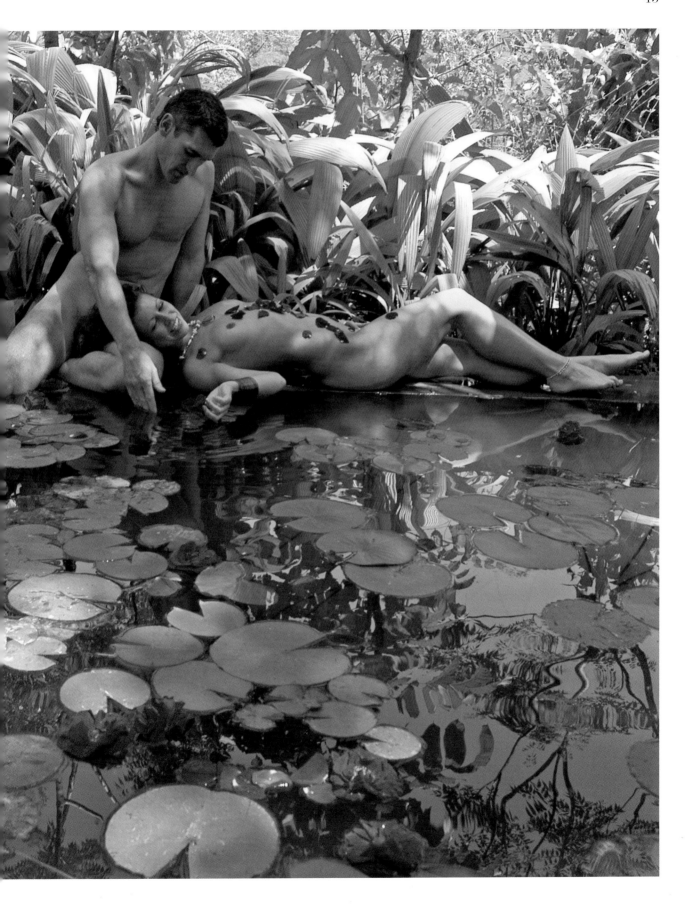

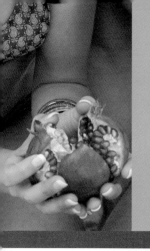

The Kama Sutra revels in sensory pleasures: food, drink, scents, and music. Enlivening all your senses before lovemaking transforms it into a heightened experience of pure delight.

awakening the senses

The best lovemaking delights—and makes full use of—all your senses: the touch of a lover's fingers, the unique smell of their body, the sounds of their pleasure, the taste of their skin, the look of love in their eyes.

But it is easy to rely on one sensation to arouse you. For men it is often visual cues, while for women, touch can be a crucial source of pleasure.

Taking time to awaken all the senses, by trying the familiar in an unfamiliar way, is a liberating experience. It also adds playfulness and creativity to your relationship as you imaginatively stimulate your lover's senses.

SENSUAL PICNIC BASKET

A natural setting is perfect for a sensory stimulation exercise as the ingredients for a "sensual picnic basket" are all around you. When planning your basket, consider each of the senses in turn and prepare—without your

Juicy melons and exotic, scented fruit are the perfect ingredients for your sensual picnic basket.

partner seeing—a range of different objects for your lover to taste, touch, smell, and hear.

Taste Prepare bite-size morsels of different foods. They could be small pieces of fruit with interesting textures, such as peeled grapes, or perfumed mango or lychees. Try squares of chocolate or pieces of crystallized ginger. Make sure it is all fresh and organic. Have some water to hand as well and, for a hot day, frozen fruit juice is great too.

Sound Find natural objects in your outdoor setting to create "wild music"—pebbles to knock together, crisp twigs for snapping, dry leaves to rustle and crunch.

Touch There should be a wealth of textures from nature to choose from, wherever you are—sand to run through fingers, blades of grass to tickle over skin, drops of cool water, bark from a tree.

Smell Nature's scents are the most delicious of all: pine cones, driftwood, fresh flowers, herbs. You could also try some essential oils, dabbed onto tissues.

SENSORY TREATS

When your hamper is ready, blindfold your lover. This will enliven their other senses as well as enhancing the trust and intimacy between you.

Take your time to arouse each sense in turn.

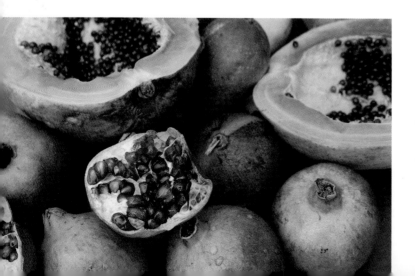

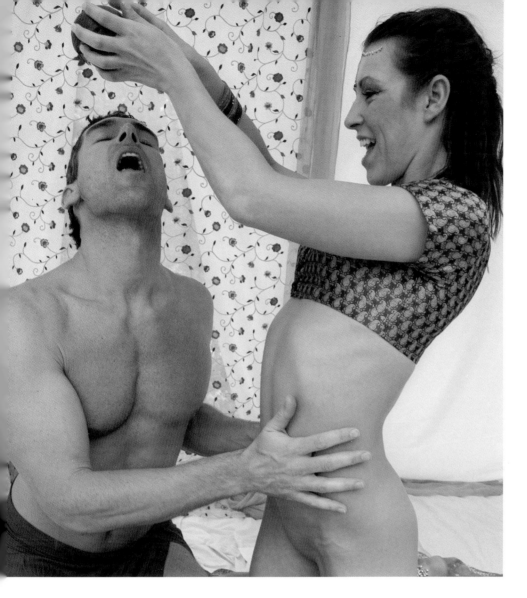

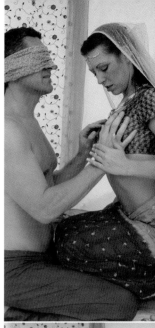

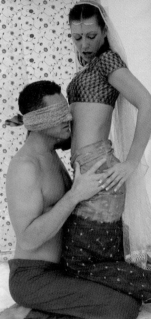

Kiss their lips then feed them morsels of food, letting them touch and smell each morsel first. Massage and nibble their ears then create different sounds around them—can they guess what they are? To awaken their sense of smell, pick up the objects and slowly waft their scents under your lover's nose. Do they bring up any memories? Allow time between the scents for the sense of smell to recover.

Now play with different textures. Finally, hold up something beautiful, such as a flower or shell, so it is the first thing your lover sees when you remove the blindfold. Or lead them to a spot where they'll get a different view of the landscape.

EXPLORE YOUR PARTNER

An erotic variation on this sensory exercise is to treat your lover as your own personal sensual picnic hamper. Ask them to blindfold you, then explore their body using different senses in turn. Smell every inch of their skin, explore it using your fingertips and, finally, use your tongue.

Heighten and arouse your senses by playing together before you make love. Using a blindfold can intensify your sense of touch.

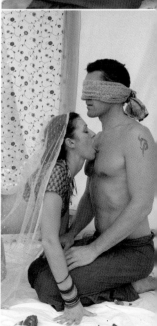

Love talk, gifts, shared leisure activities— the Kama Sutra recognizes all these as important aspects of courtship. Today they remain an essential preliminary to seduction and are valuable whether you are new lovers or life-long partners.

the art of wooing

The Kama Sutra advises that lovers spend time with each other talking, eating, and gently touching before lovemaking.

Vatsyayana recognized the importance of preparing the mind—as well as the body—for love. Wooing might seem an outdated concept in the age of speed-dating, but the joys of seduction, however long you and your lover have been in the relationship, never fade. Vatsyayana, describing a typical seduction scene of the time, recommends talking "suggestively" as a wonderful way to build up your anticipation (see panel opposite). If your

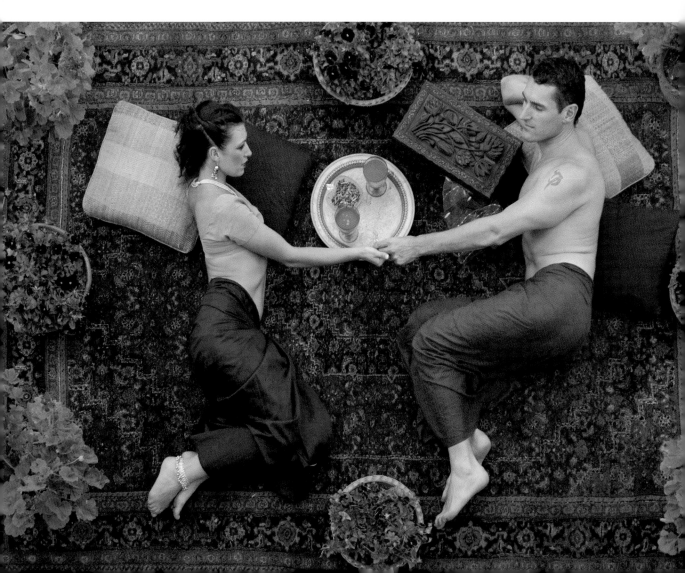

"In the pleasure-room, decorated with flowers, and fragrant with perfumes, attended by his friends and servants, the citizen should receive the woman, who will come bathed and dressed, and will invite her to take refreshment and to drink freely. He should then seat her on his left side, and holding her hair, and touching also the end and knot of her garment, he should gently embrace her with his right arm. They should then carry on an amusing conversation on various subjects, and may also talk suggestively of things which would be considered as coarse, or not to be mentioned generally in society."

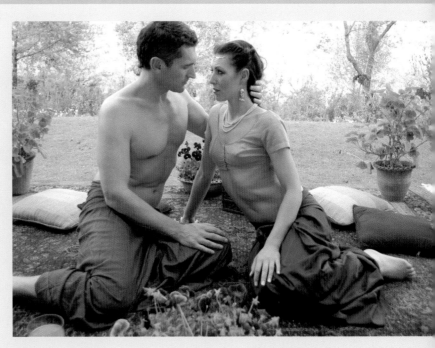

outdoor rendezvous is being planned in advance, make the most of the excitement of thinking about where you are going, and what you would like to do—and have done to you—when you get there.

Share your fantasy romantic outdoor scenarios and be imaginative in how you communicate. Leave love notes and send each other suggestive text messages and emails: the aphrodisiac power of erotic talk cannot be overestimated.

LOVERS' GIFTS

Vatsyayana suggests that, when a man is courting a woman, "he should procure for her such playthings as may be hardly known to other girls," and also recommends bouquets of flowers, clothing, and jewelry. These are still acknowledged as the classic gifts of seduction. But while giving is an important part of wooing, gifts need not be material objects.

A gift can be verbal, simply saying, "I love you" or "You look gorgeous" to your partner, for example, or noticing something different about them—a flattering haircut or new clothing item—and commenting on it. In a long-term relationship, this acts as a welcome reminder that your partner is still "seeing" and appreciating you. Simple gifts, such as cooking your lover's favorite meal (and clearing away afterward) are treats that show thoughtfulness.

Spending time together, sharing pastimes and simple unhurried pleasures are among the greatest gifts you can give in a relationship. This is even more important if you have children, to remind yourselves that you are lovers as well as parents. If so, hire a reliable baby-minder occasionally, and resist the temptation to spend the time catching up on sleep. Instead, court each other anew, rekindling the early spark of your love affair.

"When a boy has thus begun to woo the girl he loves, he should spend his time with her and amuse her with various games and diversions fitted for their age and acquaintanceship, such as picking and collecting flowers, making garlands of flowers, playing the parts of members of a fictitious family, cooking food, playing with dice, playing with cards…"

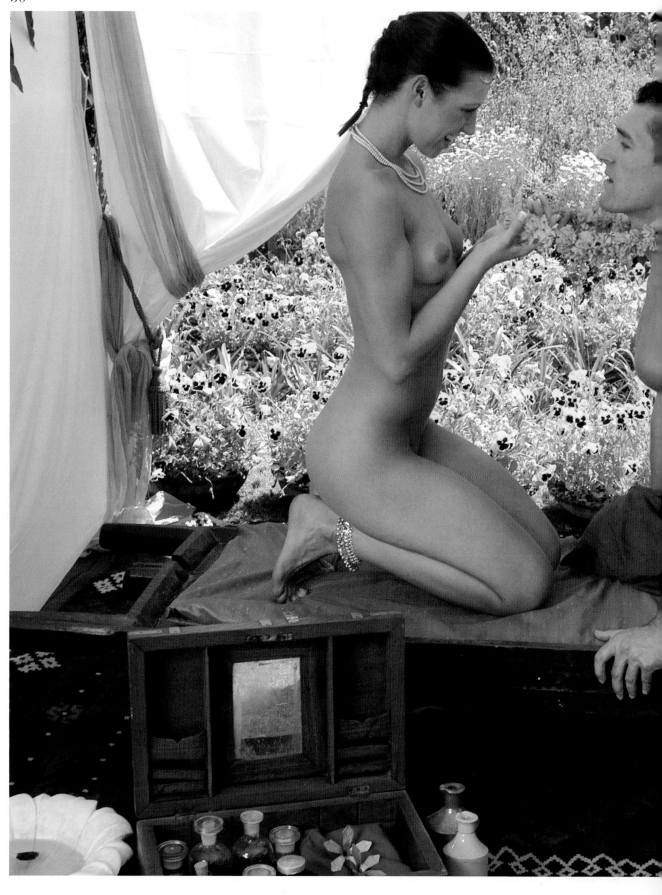

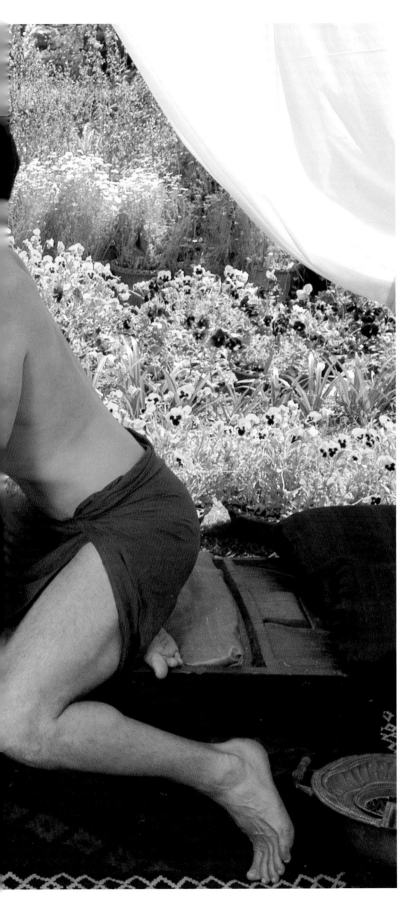

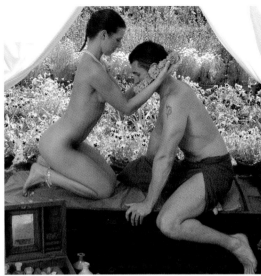

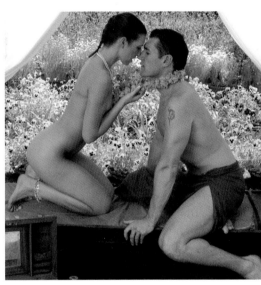

*Woo your lover with
words and gestures,
drawing them closer to
you in the lead-up to
lovemaking.*

CHAPTER 4

tantalizing touch

The Kama Sutra describes the seduction of a virgin bride in which her new husband woos her for many nights before intercourse takes place. He gradually moves from embraces to caressing her breasts, and then strokes the whole body of his young wife, before beginning to teach her the sexual arts.

PROLONG THE MOMENT

While you and your lover may not choose to extend your making out over a number of nights, the principle of "slow is better" still holds true for building up anticipation and arousal.

Follow Vatsyayana's advice and take your time to gently arouse each other to boiling point. From a simple embrace in which you express all the tenderness you feel for your lover, to using tantalizing touch to explore and awaken every inch of your partner's body, prolonging the tension of the sexual build-up is an art in itself that encompasses more than our usual notion of "foreplay."

Loving touch is one of the most erotic ways to arouse delicious sensations of anticipation, and the Kama Sutra has lots of suggestions for awakening the entire body through embracing, kissing, stroking, and scratching.

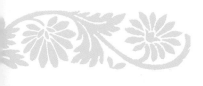

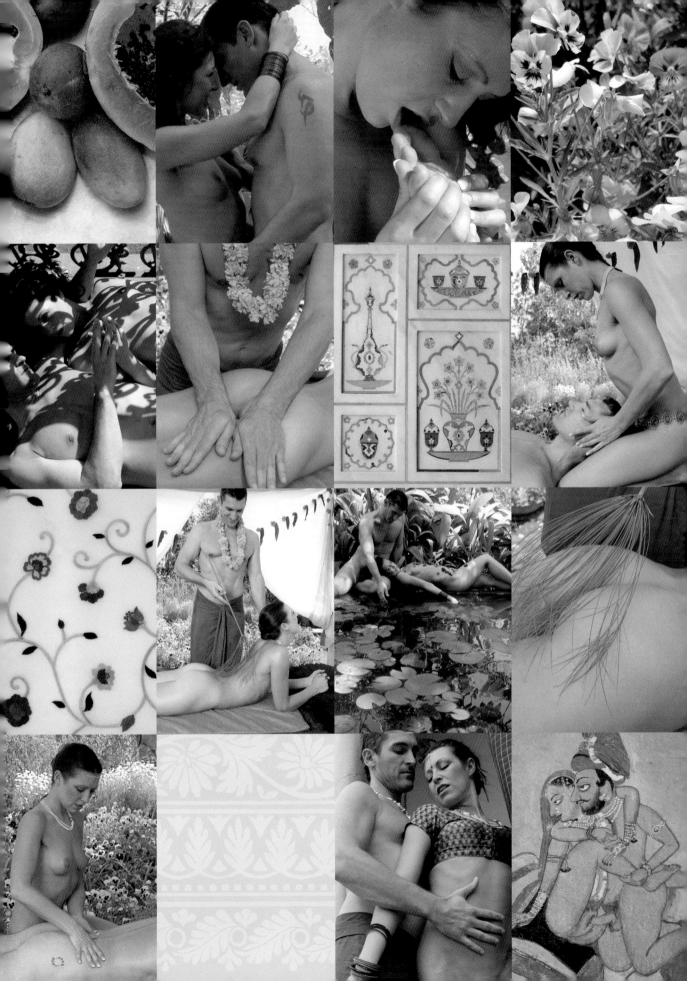

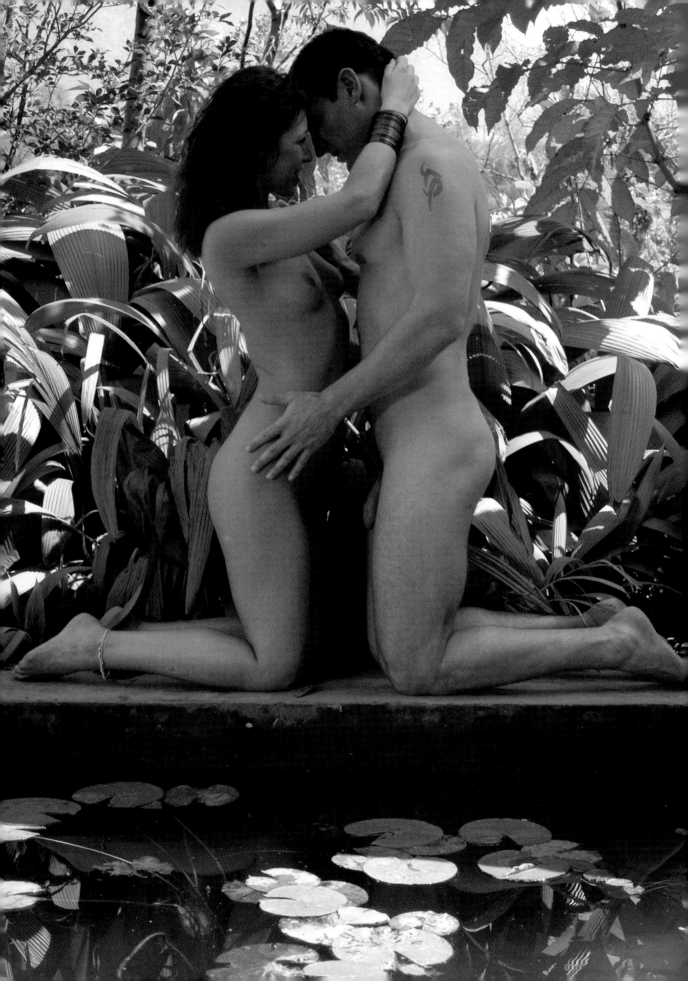

A simple embrace is a moment of stillness. Wrap your arms around your lover and you express your feelings with your whole body and heart.

the embrace

Simply holding your partner lovingly is an act of great tenderness. Whether it's a fully clothed, reassuringly lingering hug, an arousing prelude to greater passion, or perhaps the warm, satisfied cuddle of post-coital bliss, being in your lover's arms inevitably increases your feelings intimacy.

Vatsyayana understood this and devoted a whole chapter of the Kama Sutra to the embraces that indicate "the mutual love of a man and woman who have come together." It may seem a tame subject for a book better known for its acrobatic sexual positions, but the power of the embrace lies in its simplicity.

A TENDER TOUCH

Next time your lover is tense, try holding them calmly in your arms in a strong embrace and feel their tension begin to gradually slip away as their shoulders relax and drop and their body becomes softer. This kind of tender touch, which comes without demands or expectations, nurtures the connection between you and your partner.

Embraces can also express deep desire and passion—it's the intention you bring to an embrace that gives it its meaning—but at its heart is always a sense of togetherness.

MELTING AND MERGING

As part of slowed-down lovemaking, the hug is invaluable. A "melting embrace" in which you hold each other with your whole bodies touching for a long time, is great for gently

"tuning in" to each other before lovemaking. As you hold each other, let your breathing harmonize, bringing your awareness into the moment, and enjoy the love connection between you.

Take time to hold your partner and make every embrace matter. If you are usually the first to break an embrace, then next time you are hugging and are about to let go, hold on for a few moments longer and let your love express itself in your encircling arms.

EMBRACING

"When a man under some pretext or other goes in front or alongside of a woman and touches her body with his own, it is called the 'touching embrace.'

When a woman in a lonely place bends down, as if to pick up something, and pierces, as it were, a man sitting or standing, with her breasts, and the man in return takes hold of them, it is called a 'piercing embrace.'

When two lovers are walking slowly together, either in the dark, or in a place of public resort, or in a lonely place, and rub their bodies against each other, it is called a 'rubbing embrace.'
When on the above occasion one of them presses the other's body forcibly against a wall or pillar, it is called a 'pressing embrace.'"

Vatsyayana's observations on the variety of embraces, distinguished by their setting or intention, demonstrate the pleasures of this simple human touch.

A beautifully intimate foreplay gift to your lover is to take the time to investigate their body inch by inch, from the crown of their head to the tips of their toes, and awaken their entire body through your touch.

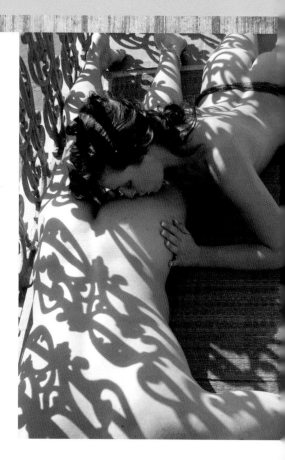

exploring your lover's body

According to Eastern sexual wisdom, the whole body is an erogenous zone—once it is awakened by an imaginative touch. Get to know every inch of your lover's body as they lie back, relax, and surrender to the pleasure of being adored.

Part of the fun of doing this is to find those unexpected hotspots so, to begin with, avoid the obvious contenders—genitals and nipples—and focus your attention on those areas you might not normally think of as sexual. Some starting points are:

• Trace every detail of your lover's back with gentle caresses and soft circles and then bring your lips very close to the skin to blow along the length of it.

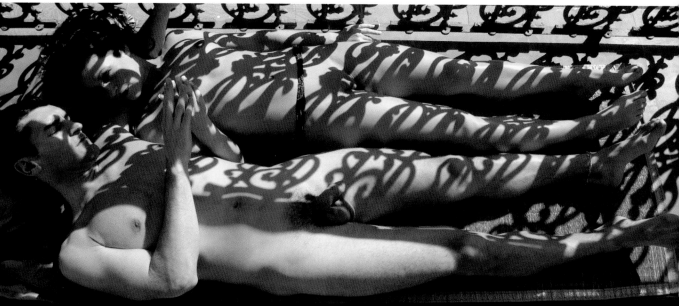

*Tantalizing
Touch*

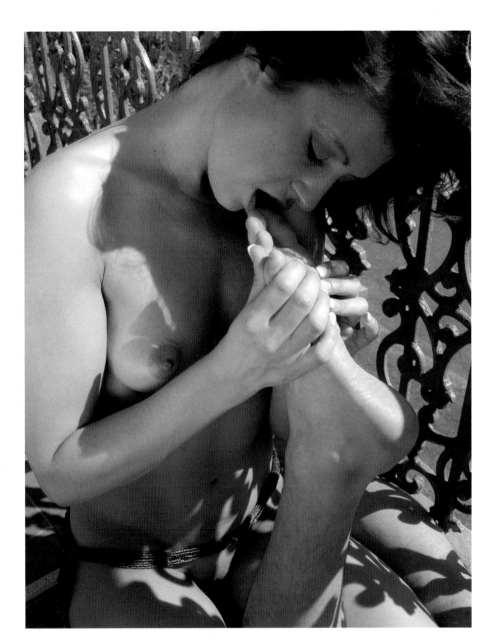

VARY YOUR TOUCH

Use hands and fingers to stroke, knead, press, and enfold. Fingertips can circle, trace, caress, and scratch—and use a light pressure to make the skin tingle. Keep the movements slow and continuous.

Use your mouth and tongue and intersperse feathery kisses with wide open caresses. Try blowing, biting (gently!), and sucking.

Make use of your entire body: try gently tweaking and circling with your toes, and stroking calves and kneading buttocks with your feet. If you have long hair, sweep it lightly over your lover's skin.

• Knead and gently shake the buttocks, and kiss along the crease where each cheek meets the top of the thigh.

• Explore the shape of the hand and forearm using the tips of your nails, and run your tongue all the way along the inner arm from the wrist to the elbow crease.

• Play with the toes, gently pulling and pressing each in turn and blow into the creases between the toes.

• Caress their head, slowly stroking it with your fingertips, and run your fingers through their hair.

SCRATCHING

"When love becomes intense, pressing with the nails or scratching the body with them is practiced."

Vatsyayana talks about scratching your lover—to the extent of leaving marks—with an enthusiasm that might seem surprising today. These "marks of love" remind one of the person who made them, and there are different scratches that can be used:

• Sounding: pressing, leaving only a small indentation

• Half moon: a curved mark made with one nail

• Circle: when two half moon marks are made opposite each other

• Line: a straight mark, when the fingernail is drawn across the skin

• Tiger's nail or claw: a curved line

• Peacock's foot: a mark made by all five nails

• Leaf of a blue lotus: marks made in a leaf pattern

Even gentle scratching will arouse the skin. Start off very lightly when you use your fingernails and be guided by their response.

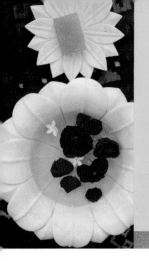

A massage is the ultimate form of relaxation so, in order to attain a state of complete bliss, your setting needs to be comfortable, warm, and as secluded as possible.

preparing for an outdoor massage

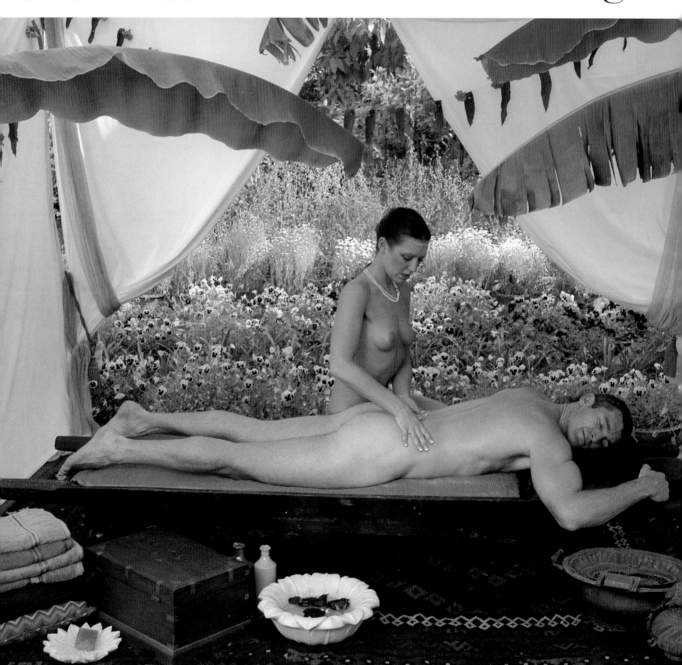

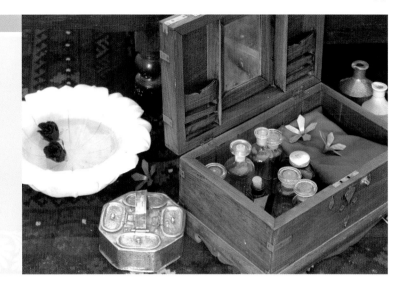

A HOME HAVEN

Close to home, such as in your outdoor boudoir, prepare a soft area for your lover to lie on, and think about how to enhance every sensual aspect of the setting. If you are near trees, try hanging sheets of silk above your partner that will move in the breeze and gently stroke their body. Deep, rich colors will add to the visual experience. You can have very gentle music playing or wind-chimes, or simply be attuned to nature's sounds such as birdsong or crickets chirruping.

A DISTANT LOCATION

A romantic outdoor setting that is further from home requires a little more work, but the added sensual nature of the setting—perhaps the sound of a running stream or the smell of the sea—will enhance the experience.

Privacy is crucial. In order to relax completely, you need to ensure you won't be disturbed by hikers. Nudity is more comfortable on a warm day but, in hot weather, avoid sunburn and find a shady spot. Under the canopy of a large tree is ideal, providing a beautiful backdrop for the massager-receiver as they lie supine. Allow enough space to move all around their body.

MASSAGE INGREDIENTS

Prepare a basket containing everything you will need. The essentials are:
• Something soft for the massage-receiver to lie on (you could make a mattress out of blankets covered with a sheet or towel or, if you are camping, try a camping mat and sleeping bag covered with a towel)
• Towels (plenty—they can also be used as support for knees, elbows, and ankles)
• A pillow or rolled towel to support the receiver's head
• Something soft to go under the massage-giver's knees
• Oils (ideally in light, spill-proof plastic bottles)
• A soft wrap (as an emergency cover-up and to allow the massage-receiver to be warm and comfortable after the massage without having to dress)
• Water to drink afterward

OILS

Preparing oils for massage is a sensual experience in itself. You will need a carrier (or base) oil to help your hands glide—try almond or grape seed. Add some essential oils for fragrance. These should only ever be used in dilute form. Add six drops of essential oil to two tablespoons of carrier oil and you should have the right quantity for a full body massage.

Essential oils with aphrodisiac qualities include sandalwood, ylang ylang, rose, and jasmine. Lavender is a great all-round oil and is wonderful for general relaxation, while neroli is especially sensual. Experiment to find the combination that delights you both.

There's always room for intuition, imagination and spontaneity with an outdoor sensual massage, but learning some basic strokes will get you off to a good, confident start.

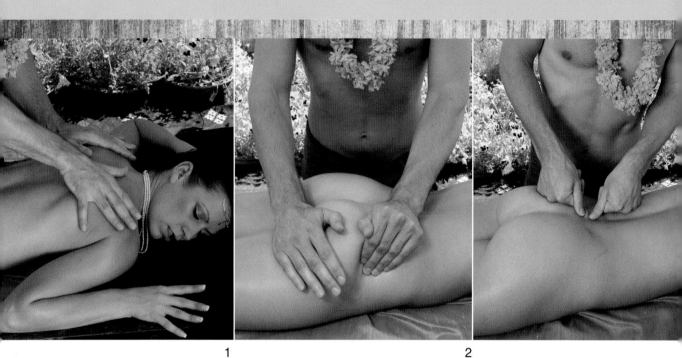

1   2

massage strokes

Basic massage strokes are simple to learn and can be put to good use when touching your lover at other times, too. When you need to break contact with your lover's body, to replenish the oil or change stroke, do it as smoothly and gently as possible so that they barely notice.

1. Effleurage

This is the starting stroke. Effleurage involves wide sweeping strokes of the hand that glide across the body, spreading the oil and seeking out areas of tension. After effleurage, squeeze along muscles such as the calves with your hand in the V shape, with thumb and forefinger spread. Push toward the heart with a firm pressure, squeezing your hand to enclose the muscle.

2. Petrissage

When a deeper touch is required, petrissage is ideal. Knead the flesh with a squeezing, rolling, and lifting action, moving your hands alternately. This feels great around the waist and on the buttocks.

3. Friction

Areas of deep tension are released using friction. Lean your weight onto the pads of your thumb with a slight circling motion to apply pressure on a specific area.

GETTING READY

Make sure you are both happy to give and receive a massage. Bear in mind that any tiredness or resentment will be felt through your hands. It's a good idea to tune into each other first by breathing gently together and eye-gazing.

Giving a massage can be physically demanding, so before you begin, stretch to relax your neck and shoulder muscles, and then give your hands a shake. When massaging, lean in using your weight, rather than muscle tension, to exert pressure so that the movements come from your whole body and flow through your arms, rather than pushing with them. Keep movements rhythmic and avoid straining when reaching or exerting pressure.

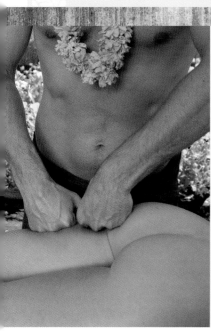

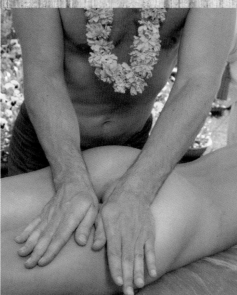

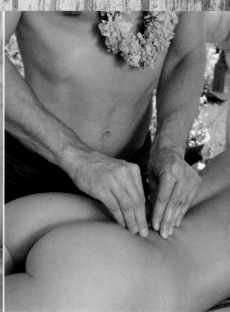

4

5

6

4. *Knuckling*

This is good for fleshy areas such as the buttocks and thighs—press down and twist with your hand bent into a loose fist while moving the knuckles.

5. *Heeling*

Stretching out your hand and lifting up your palm and fingers, use the heel of your hand to push muscle away from you in a deep, penetrating, circling stroke, which is ideal for thigh muscles and buttocks.

6. *Fingertips*

Use your fingertips for light, delicate caresses of the face and little fingertip-steps along the length of the back.

NATURAL VARIATIONS

Be imaginative and use the nature around you. Smooth pebbles make a wonderful massage tool.

Try warming them in the sun first, or cooling them off in water, for a sensational effect.

A sheaf of long grass, big leaves, or flowers are great for tickling and stroking. Feathers—traditionally peacock feathers in the Kama Sutra age—have much erotic potential.

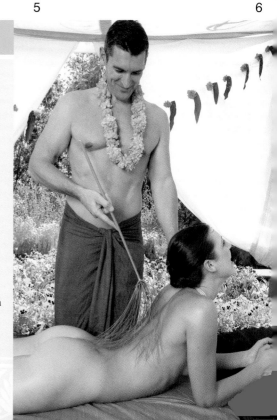

Once you discover what your lover likes most you can devise a tailor-made massage just for them. Devoting your undivided attention to every part of your lover's body is a wonderful gift.

giving a sensual massage

Individual sections can be enjoyed on their own when you don't have time for a full massage.

THE BACK

Warm some oil in your hands and glide your hands up your lover's back, either side of the spine. Work upward and outward in a fan shape. Spread more oil onto the buttocks, and knead them with the heels of your hands.

Moving down to the back of the legs, use sweeping strokes with a steady rhythm. With your hand in a V shape, squeeze along the calf muscles with thumb and forefinger. Work on both legs at the same time, or start on the calf of one as your other hand reaches the buttock of the other. Be careful with the back of the knee area.

HEAD, FACE, AND NECK

Ask your lover to lie on their back and then kneel either side of their head. Use delicate strokes to ease tension in head, face, and neck muscles. Press slowly at the back of the neck, and gently roll the head from side to side to ease tension.

Knead the scalp and run your fingers through their hair, tweaking tufts, and making small circling movements with your thumbs. Massage the face with outward strokes and pay special attention to eye and jaw area. Trace circles around their temples, smooth the cheeks, and then place your thumbs in the center of your lover's forehead and gradually draw them apart. Now massage the earlobes with little squeezing and pulling movements.

EROTIC VARIATION

An erotic option is to start at the head and work down toward the abdomen, then from feet to abdomen, so that the massage finishes at the genital area.

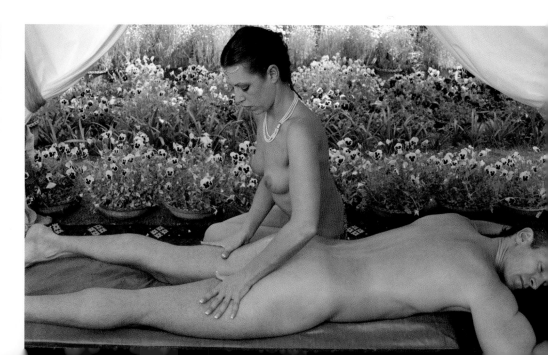

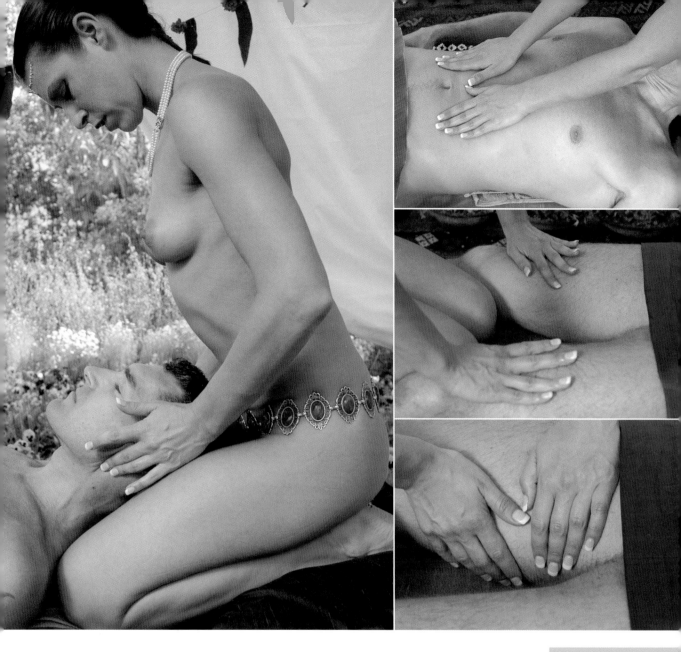

ARMS AND CHEST

Moving around to the side, use effleurage on the arms, working along the length of the forearm muscles. Squeeze, followed by fingertip caresses. Then work from elbow to shoulder. Massage each hand in turn, using your thumb to work on the knuckles and joints and gently pull each finger in turn. Caress the palms of the hands and gently squeeze and roll the wrists. Use gliding effleurage strokes between and over the breasts or pectoral muscles to release tension in the chest.

ABDOMEN AND LEGS

As you move down to the abdomen, keep your touch warm and gentle, and let your hands rest on the center of the stomach for a few moments. Then circle your hands over the belly, in a clockwise direction.

Working along the fronts of the legs, from ankles to hips, use a petrissage stroke for deeper pressure on the thighs and a much lighter touch to circle the kneecap.

FOCUS ON THE FEET

Hold the feet softly for a few moments of grounding then smooth over the tops of each foot with your thumbs. Play with the toes, gently pulling, stretching, and shaking each in turn. Use a light pressure around the instep and, as you finish with each foot, again enfold it lovingly in both your hands.

GROUNDING CONCLUSION

Feathery strokes across the whole body are an uplifting way to finish, then rest your hands lightly on your lover's body for a few moments.

CHAPTER 5

the art of oral erotics

The mouth is one of the most sensitive parts of the body. Kissing, sucking, licking, blowing, nibbling, biting… the possibilities for erotic arousal—using just the mouth and tongue—are endless.

KISSING MASTER CLASS

From the first kiss, which marks the transition from friendship to something more, to the deep kisses of passionate lovers, the barriers between you dissolve when two mouths meet. So much is expressed in a kiss. The Kama Sutra recognizes this with a whole array of different kinds of kisses to try.

But the Kama Sutra "way of the mouth" goes far beyond simple mouth-to-mouth kissing. Exploring every inch of your lover's skin with just mouth and tongue is a highly erotic game to play during foreplay. The Kama Sutra also has advice for lovers who are tempted by the fiercer pleasures of biting.

MOUTH AND TONGUE TECHNIQUES

Oral sex is perhaps one of the most arousing uses of the kiss in lovemaking. Variety is the key to great oral sex, and in this chapter you can discover exciting and erotic techniques to stimulate your lover through "congress of the crow," fellatio, and cunnilingus.

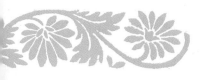

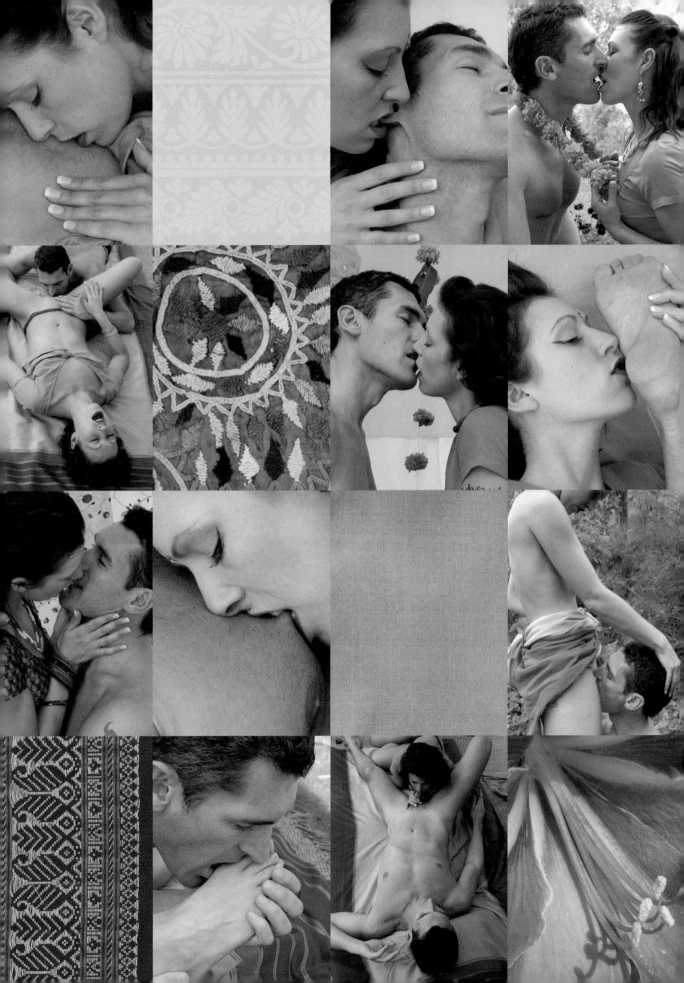

Kissing is a vital way to connect intimately with your lover throughout lovemaking—before, during, and after. For Kama Sutra lovers, the "way of the mouth" is an art in itself.

AWAKENING

"When a woman looks at the face of her lover while he is asleep and kisses it to show her intention or desire, it is called a 'kiss that kindles love.'
When a lover coming home late at night, kisses his beloved, who is asleep on her bed, in order to show her his desire, it is called a 'kiss that awakens.'"

the kiss

The mouth has an immense capacity for giving and receiving pleasure. It is packed full of nerve endings, and combines the properties of the penis (the tongue) with the vulva (the mouth and lips). According to the ancient Eastern path of Tantra, a woman's upper lip is connected directly to the clitoris by a special nerve channel.

From the first, tentative kiss of new lovers to love-filled post-coital caresses, the way you kiss expresses so much. Gentle, light, feathery kisses evoke tenderness, while deep kissing expresses intimacy and urgent, erotic energy.

Vatsyayana sets out different types of kisses, from the "nominal" kiss—when a girl lightly touches the mouth of her lover with her own—to the intense "fighting of the tongues."

Kissing is an essential part of foreplay, triggering arousal and passion. But the joy of a long, sexy kiss should be enjoyed at any time, especially in long-term relationships, and not just as a prelude to sex.

KINDLING KISSES

Kissing can also be a way to gently awaken your sleeping lover and tenderly indicate your desire for them, as the Kama Sutra suggests

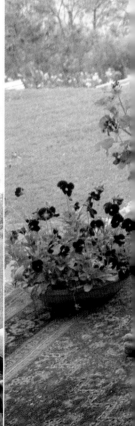

Kissing can be teasing, playful, or passionate and the full repertoire of kissing has a place in sensual lovemaking.

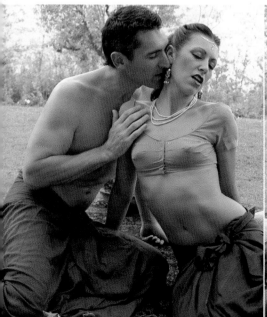
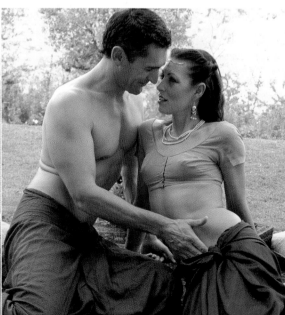

beautifully with two "kindling kisses" (see 'Awakening' panel, page 66).

SURPRISE KISS

Next time, surprise your partner and, instead of that quick kiss, express all your love for them with your mouth and tongue—but without words…

• Suck your lover's thumbs and fingers and lick the skin between the fingers.
• Delicately lick and suck your partner's mouth, taking upper or lower lips between your own for gentle sucking and licking.
• Gently nip the upper or lower lip with your teeth.
• Kiss around the mouth, and the upper and lower lips in turn. Be delicate with your tongue, retreating and advancing, darting and circling.
• Alternate between hard, urgent kisses and soft, feathery ones.

SENSATIONAL KISSING

Experiment with different temperatures: use ice cold water or a warm drink and dip your tongue into each in turn before kissing, teasing your lover with the contrasting sensations.

THE KAMA SUTRA KISSING GAME

"As regards kissing, a wager may be laid as to which will get hold of the lips of the other first. If the woman loses, she should pretend to cry, should keep her lover off by shaking her hands, and turn away… saying, 'let another wager be laid.' If she loses this a second time, she should appear doubly distressed, and when her lover is off his guard or asleep, she should get hold of his lower lip, and hold it in her teeth, so that it should not slip away, and then she should laugh, make a loud noise, deride him, dance about, and say whatever she likes in a joking way…"

Vatsyayana's description in the Kama Sutra of a playful kissing game between lovers.

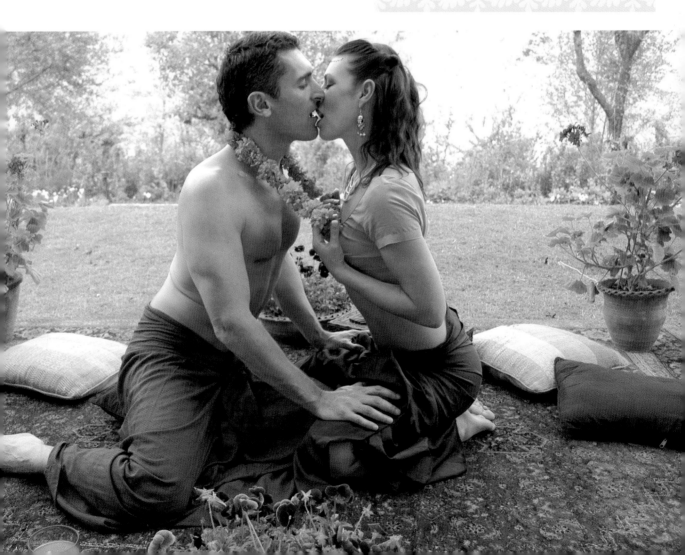

Caressing with mouth alone is a highly erotic way to begin lovemaking. Make it delicious for you both by starting with light kisses, slowly tracing the contours of your lover's body with your lips.

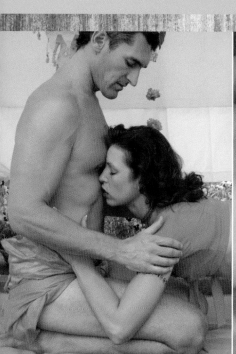
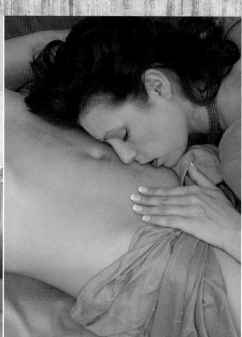
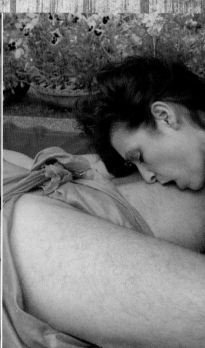

the way of the mouth

CARESS THE CURVES

Soft kisses across the belly can be wonderfully sensual, while delicate kisses on the inner thigh are tantalizingly tingly for men and women alike. Try the nape of the neck—blowing lightly on the soft hairs there—and run your tongue along the line of the shoulders. Seek out areas of soft skin to nuzzle with your mouth—the crease of the elbow, armpit, small of the back—and trace wet kisses around larger areas of your lover's body.

Nibble earlobes and experiment by gently exploring your lover's inner ear with your tongue. But be warned: it might drive your lover absolutely wild, or could arouse fits of giggles rather than moans of pleasure—it's not to everyone's taste!

Play with your lover's nipples with your lips, tongue, and teeth. A man's nipples respond to a teasing touch just as well as a woman's and are often ignored.

BITE OF LOVE

As you increase the pressure of your kisses from light to firm, you may be tempted to use your teeth lightly, too. Vatsyayana advises that "all the places that can be kissed are also the places that can be bitten, except the upper lip, the interior of the mouth, and the eyes."

A bite that leaves a red mark can be painful

"Kissing is of four kinds: moderate, contracted, pressed, and soft, according to the different parts of the body which are kissed, for different kinds of kisses are appropriate for different parts of the body."

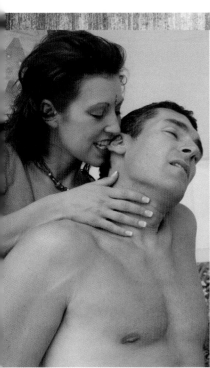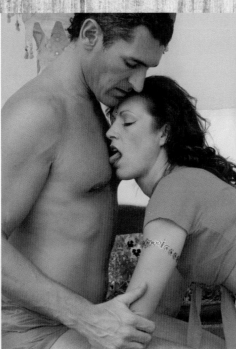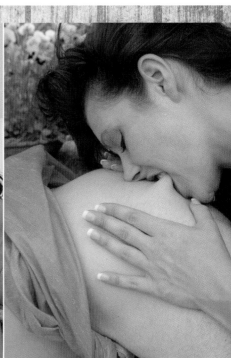

so go gently, be aware of your lover's pain threshold, and choose a little light nibbling on fleshy areas such as the buttocks, rather than sinking your teeth in. The Kama Sutra gives detailed advice on the kinds of biting that can be pleasurably performed. These include:
• Hidden bite—shown only by the excessive redness of the skin
• Swollen bite—the skin is pressed down on both sides
• Point—a small portion of the skin is bitten with two teeth only
• Line of points—small portions of the skin are bitten with all the teeth
• Coral and jewel—bringing together the teeth (jewel) and lips (coral)
• Broken cloud—marks on the breasts that consist of unequal risings in a circle, and that

come from the space between the teeth
• Biting of a boar—marks on breasts and shoulders that consist of many broad rows of marks near to one another

THE KAMA SUTRA BITING GAME

"When a man bites a woman forcibly, she should angrily do the same to him with double force. Thus a 'point' should be returned with a 'line of points,' and a 'line of points' with a 'broken cloud,' and if she be excessively chafed … should take hold of her lover by the hair, and bend his head down, and kiss his lower lip, and then, being intoxicated with love, she should shut her eyes and bite him in various places."

The Kama Sutra a "biting game," which may sound too violent for modern-day tastes.

Oral sex is the most intimate of sexual acts, and one of the most erotically satisfying. It is also an act of "honoring" in which you worship the sacred in your lover.

oral sex: divine pleasures

MATTERS OF SIZE

Vatsyayana classifies lovers according to size of genitals. A man is a hare, bull, or horse, according to the length of his lingam. A women is a deer, mare, or elephant, depending on the depth of her yoni. The Kama Sutra recommends "equal union" between lovers of corresponding sizes for the greatest satisfaction but suggests positions that lovers of "unequal" size can enjoy to accommodate their differences.

SEXUAL SYMBOLISM

In the Kama Sutra, the male and female genitals are regarded as sacred and should be treated with reverence. The vulva is honored as the gateway to life, the most divine part of a woman's body. "Yoni" is the Sanskrit word for the female sexual organs and means "sacred place," the source of all life and universal bliss. It symbolizes the female energy of the great goddess and was worshipped in early cultures with "yoni goddesses"—the Venus figures with exaggerated vulvas that appear in some of the earliest known pieces of art.

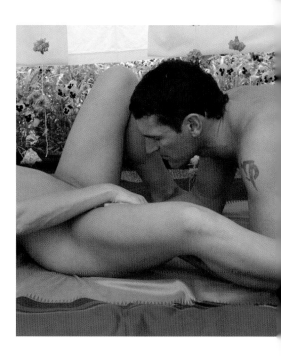

POWER AND FERTILITY

The erect phallus represents male sexual power and fertility and, in India, symbolizes the male energy of the god Shiva, and is known by the Sanskrit term "lingam." Sculptures of the erect lingam can be found in Hindu temples, where it is worshipped as an emblem of generation and recreation. These representations of lingams often have a yoni at the base to show the inseparability of male and female energy.

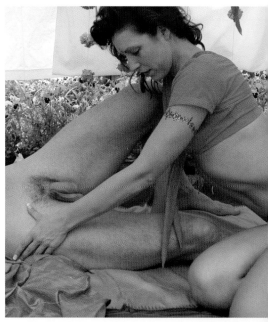

"When a man and woman lie down in an inverted order, that is, with the head of one toward the feet of the other, and carry on this congress, it is called congress of a crow."

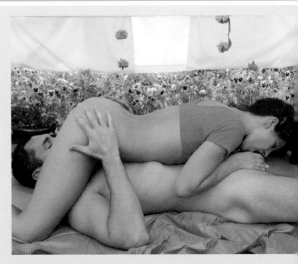

"Congress of a crow" is Vatsyayana's term for mutual oral sex, or the "69" position. An exciting way to pleasure each other, lying down with the woman on top is visually stimulating, but the most relaxed position for many couples is lying side-by-side, head resting on the lower thigh of your lover. This is perhaps best enjoyed as an arousing interlude during foreplay rather than as the main course as it can lead to the "worst of both worlds" with neither partner able to fully immerse themselves in their own enjoyment or concentrate on pleasuring their lover.

Be careful, too, of getting over-excited in the throes of passion and accidentally biting your lover's genitals!

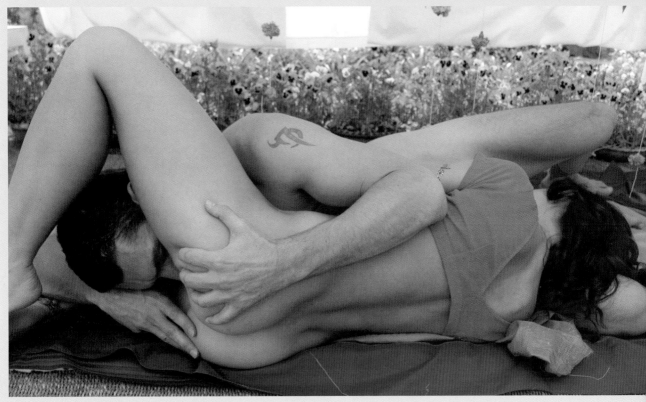

A LOVING ACT

Great oral sex requires immense trust between lovers. When you take on the perspective that the yoni and lingam are sacred and should be treated with reverence, you have already taken the act into a different dimension. Feeling that your lover is really appreciating your yoni or lingam, by looking at it lovingly, appreciating its unique shape and texture, honoring it as the essence of male or female energy, helps build up trust and reduces feelings of self-consciousness.

Watching your lover worship your yoni or lingam can be highly erotic, so try to maintain your sense of connection with each other throughout oral sex by looking toward them and making eye contact at regular intervals.

Fellatio, with its intensely erotic sensations, is highly sexually satisfying for a man. Just knowing that his lover is enthusiastic about pleasuring him orally is a great aphrodisiac in itself.

PLEASURE TIP

Remember that a lingam doesn't need to be hard in order to enjoy oral pleasuring. Letting your lover know that you appreciate his lingam in all its phases is tremendously affirming for him.

the art of fellatio

TEASING SENSATIONS

For maximum pleasure—and to ensure your lover doesn't ejaculate too soon—build up slowly and vary the sensations. A firm touch with lots of lubrication works best, so keep moistening your lips with saliva.

Tease him first, by arousing the area all around his lingam. Play with his pubic hair, massage, kiss, and lick his inner thighs, and run your tongue right along the line at the top, tantalizingly close to scrotum and lingam. Hold his scrotum, delicately pulling, tickling, and squeezing the skin (especially around the very sensitive rear of the scrotum) then take it into your mouth, running your tongue around it and flicking it with your tongue to produce delicious sensations.

FLICK AND SWIRL

Firmly holding the shaft of his lingam, begin to lick along its length, alternating between using the full width of your tongue and just the tip. Then flick your tongue around the glans, and slowly circle your lips and tongue around it. At the same time, rhythmically squeeze the shaft with your hand, or move it up and down using the lubrication you've created from your saliva. Swirl your tongue around the glans and then

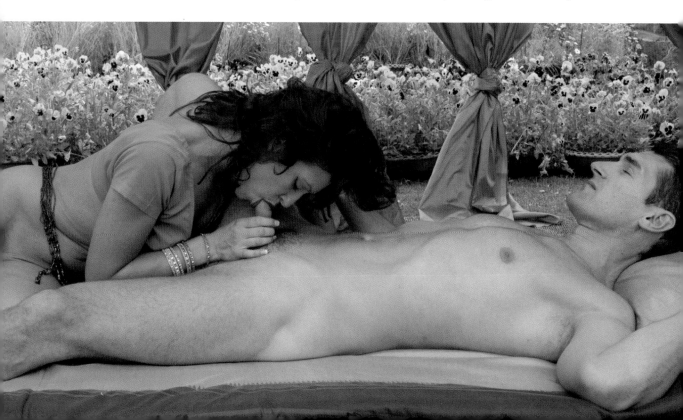

the shaft while holding him tightly in your whole mouth.

You might try relaxing the muscles at the back of your throat and swallowing a few times—an unusual and arousing sensation for him. Then take him in your mouth slowly and teasingly, gradually moving your mouth down all the way as far as you can go, and suck hard. Slowly slide your mouth all the way back up, stopping at tiny intervals to press harder with your lips and to suck.

THE MAGIC FLUTE

Alternate between using mouth and fingers—try "playing the flute." Hold the base firmly so that the skin is pulled down, and "corkscrew" your finger up and down the shaft. Squeeze, pinch, and nibble the most sensitive spot just below the glans. When your hands aren't busy on his lingam, caress his thighs or buttocks and cup and play with his testicles.

As his arousal peaks, full stroking movements—imitating intercourse—are usually preferred with firm hand or mouth and a definite rhythm. Men should be careful not to thrust too deeply into their lover's mouth, and to give warning when they are about to climax. As he comes, try flicking your tongue across the tip and stroke the shaft with your hand.

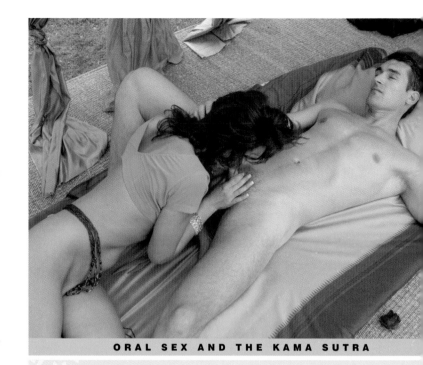

ORAL SEX AND THE KAMA SUTRA

The Kama Sutra has imaginative suggestions for "mouth congress," including:

- Nominal congress—the lingam is softly and gently caressed by the mouth
- Sucking a mango fruit—the lingam is fiercely sucked and kissed with about half of it held in the mouth
- Pressing inside—the lingam is given long deep sucks with the whole of the mouth, then slid out again

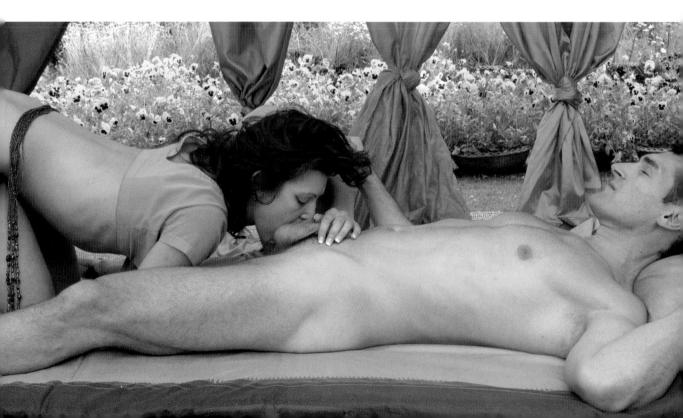

Oral sex on a woman—cunnilingus—offers intense and exciting sensations. Women who find it difficult to orgasm during intercourse often find it much easier during oral pleasuring, and may even enjoy multiple climaxes.

the art of cunnilingus

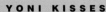

Cunnilingus is most satisfying when it is an "all-body" experience. So build up the sexual tension slowly. Begin by stroking and kissing your lover's entire body. Caress her breasts and nipples, and then slowly move down, teasingly, caressing and licking her belly, inner thighs, and the line of flesh where the top of each thigh meets the pubic area.

Take time to appreciate the sight of her yoni—and tell her so—before starting to gently kiss the whole area. Now use your tongue in one firm stroke all the way from perineum to clitoris. Kiss the lips of her yoni then use your finger and thumb to make a roll of flesh. Gently move your fingers up and down, rolling the flesh between them as you suck and nibble along the length of it.

Now hold the lips apart and play with the outer and inner lips using your mouth, lips, tongue, and fingers. Take time to inflame and arouse her before gently using your tongue or fingers to push back the hood of the clitoris, fix your lips around it and stimulate it by sucking

and flicking your tongue and nudging it with the tip of a hard and soft tongue.

GUIDE EACH OTHER

If your lover is too excited to give verbal cues, her movements may guide you as she shifts position to increase stimulation to a particular area. Stroke the tender perineum (between anus and vagina), and caress her buttocks and inner thighs.

Now use your hand and fingers to stimulate her vagina. Try stroking the inner wall with your fingers, paying special attention to the front and upper part, 1–2 inches inside, where the flesh is slightly ridged and spongy. For some women, erotic sensitivity is located in one particular zone of the anterior vaginal wall—the G-spot—while for others the pleasure zone is more spread out. Experiment!

BUILD TO A CLIMAX

As she gets more excited and approaches orgasm, keep the movements of your mouth,

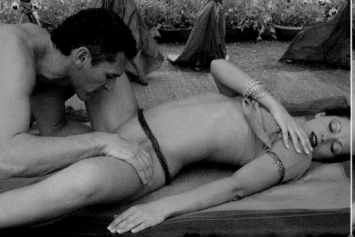

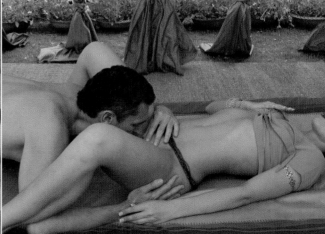

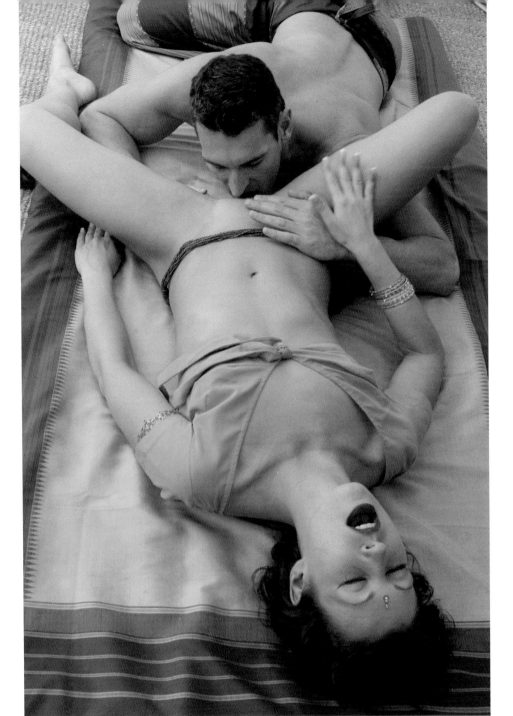

The Art of Oral Erotics

ORAL KUNG FU

Ancient Taoist masters of love called oral sex "tongue kung fu" and developed exercises for men to strengthen their tongue muscles. Let your jaw relax, then try stretching your tongue out fully, circling it first clockwise, then counterclockwise. Now reach up to your nose and down to your chin, then out to the left and then right—a regular workout that pays dividends!

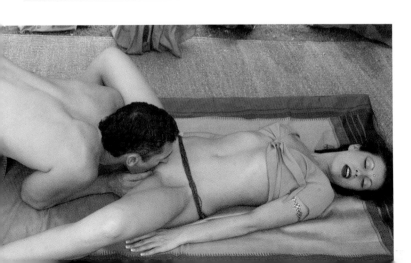

tongue, and fingers rhythmic, and be prepared to increase the pressure. At this point she may prefer you to use your fingers on her clitoris, circling with regular, steady pressure while you stimulate her vagina with your tongue. Continue to lick, suck, and stroke throughout her climax then, as she relaxes, tenderly lick the whole area from the perineum right up to her mound of Venus in long, sensual strokes of your tongue, a beautifully loving sensation.

the kama

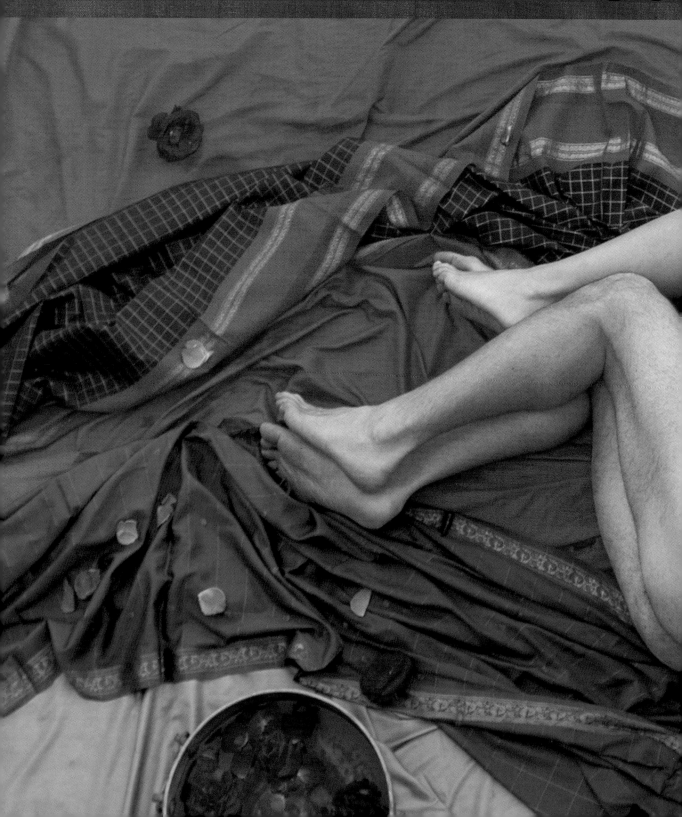

sutra

Experiment with these exciting sexual positions inspired by the Kama Sutra and discover how lovemaking can flow like a dance, moving seamlessly from one position to the next, and how the different rhythms of love can deepen and intensify your lovemaking until it becomes truly transcendent.

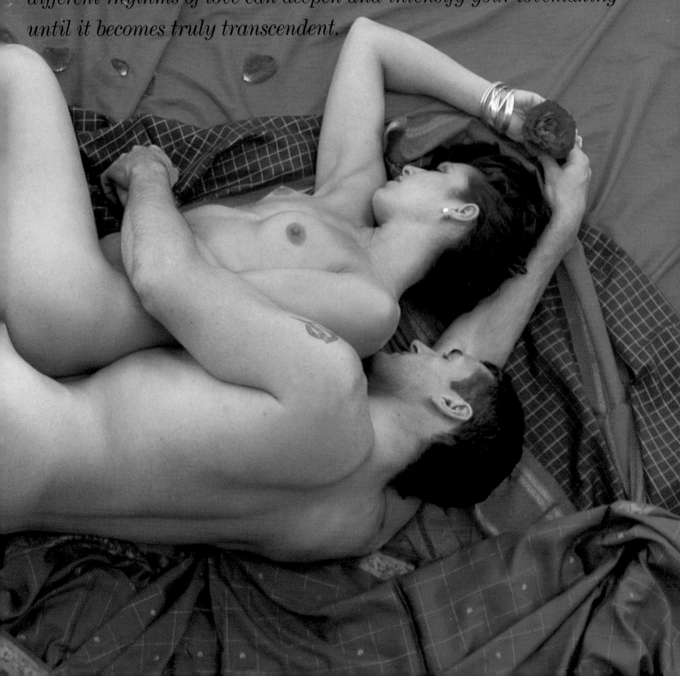

CHAPTER 6

the dance
of
love

Inspired by the classic Kama Sutra postures, this chapter offers a selection of exciting sexual positions geared toward outdoors loving. You'll find ideas for fun positions in the garden, using benches and hammocks; suggestions for lovemaking in the sea or by a stream; peaceful postures for long lazy afternoons of summer loving; and spontaneous positions for when passion overcomes you.

PLAYFUL LOVING

You'll also discover the Kama Sutra's playful nature, with lovemaking inspired by animals, and adventurous postures for more flexible lovers. Finally, a section on spiritual positions offers an insight into the sacred nature of lovemaking.

The sequences are designed to offer new ideas and inspiration, but they aren't a checklist to be ticked off—use them to discover what works for you both within your own personal dance of love. Find the true spirit of heartfelt lovemaking and trust your body's wisdom in each movement.

SHARE AND ENJOY

What is most important is the love connection between you and your partner. Having fun and sharing new experiences by trying out new ways of making love in different settings is one way to explore and deepen that connection. And if during your explorations you do discover that a certain posture takes you to new—and hitherto unimaginable—heights of erotic pleasure, then so much the better!

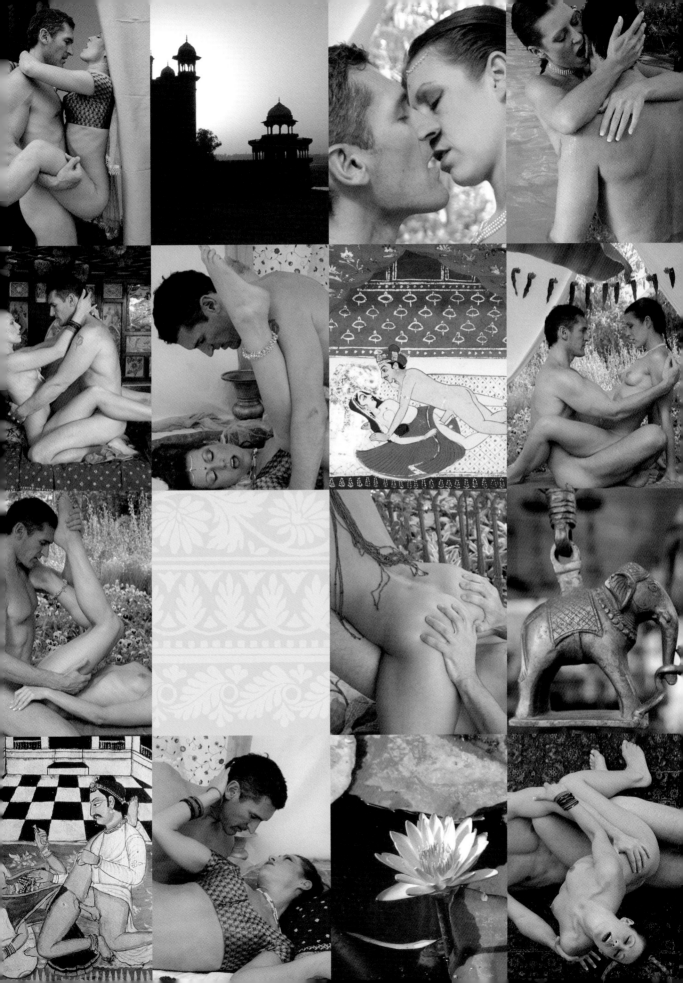

PEACEFUL POSITIONS *You lie naked with your lover, your skin warmed by the sun, with nothing to do but enjoy each other's bodies. These peaceful positions are ideal for long, languid afternoons of love.*

1 *the* blossom

This flowing set of peaceful, intimate, lying down postures offers a gentle starting point for your lovemaking, with the promise of passion. Starting in a classic man-on-top pose, the "clasping position" is a gentle, tender embrace. With the man's legs stretched straight out over the woman's, take your time to enjoy feeling the full length of your bodies pressed against each other as you gaze into each other's eyes or kiss deeply (1).

Movement is limited as you clasp, which provides a very gentle opening that blossoms into the "pressing position." Now the woman brings her thighs together under her lover to hold his lingam tightly inside her. In this position she can caress his back and grip his buttocks (2).

With the sexual energy rising, the woman raises one leg to place her thigh across the thigh of her lover, hooking her ankle under his buttock in the "twining position" (main picture). Her hands are free to reach down easily to stimulate her clitoris and caress her lover. In this position, deeper penetration is possible, and the man can press down on his hands or elbows to ease his weight off his lover's body and experiment with different angles of penetration.

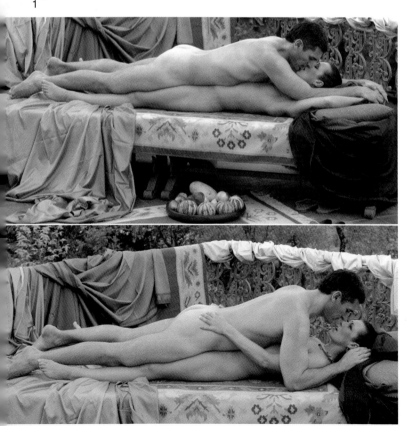

1

2

ENVELOPING EMBRACE

"When lovers embrace each other so closely that the arms and thighs of the one are encircled by the arms and thighs of the other, and are, as it were, rubbing up against them, this is called an embrace like 'the mixture of sesame seed with rice.'"

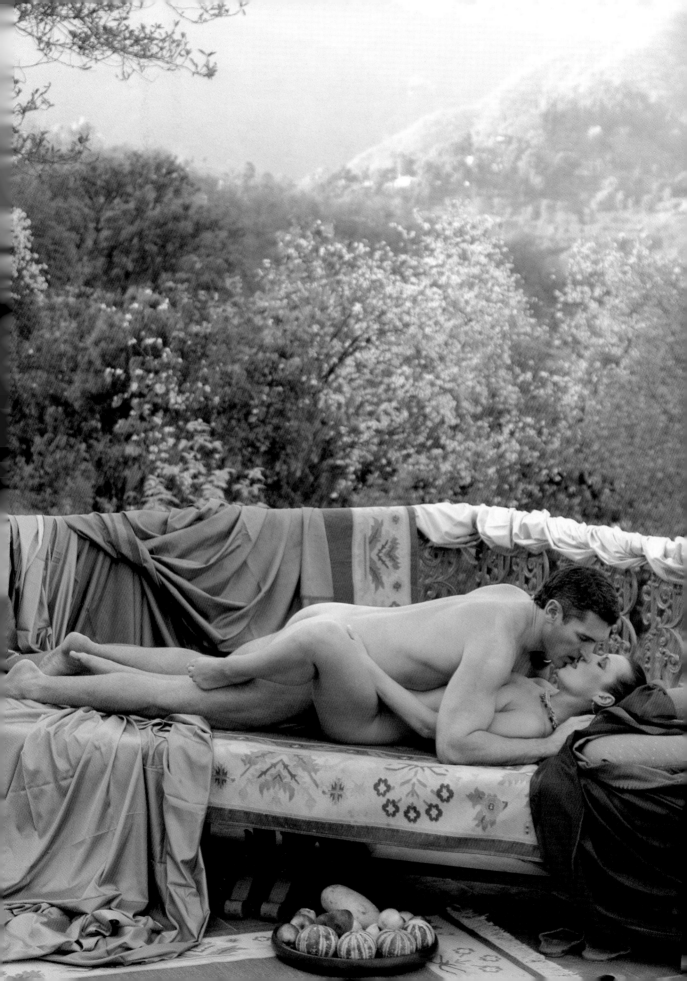

The sexual tension gradually builds up in this sequence of peaceful positions as the woman continues to recline, perhaps resting on the pillows you brought, and her lover crouches in front.

2 sweet love

The man squats, comfortably resting his weight on his feet. His lover reclines in front of him and, raising her buttocks so they rest on the insides of her partner's thighs, draws back her legs, bending her knees so that her thighs are close to her chest.

As the man enters her, she places her feet on her lover's chest (1), forming the "pressed position." From here, the man can vary the depth and direction of his thrusts as he caresses her thighs and breasts while, with her legs drawn back, the woman feels a delicious build-up of tension in her vaginal muscles.

To move into a variation—the "packed position"—which offers subtly different sensations for both lovers, the woman crosses one ankle over the other, creating a tight fit between lingam and yoni (2). Experiment with crossing and uncrossing your ankles to vary the pressure against the sides of the yoni, or the more flexible can try crossing their legs above the knee.

Now, with ankles uncrossed, the woman stretches out one leg towards the sky or along her lover's side, leaving the other bent toward her chest (3). In this highly arousing position, the man caresses his lover's legs and breasts while thrusting gently. The woman enjoys the sensation of her partner's movements against her clitoris.

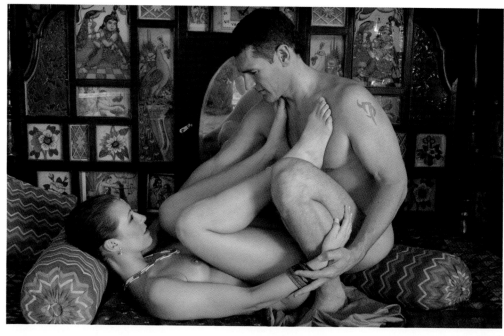

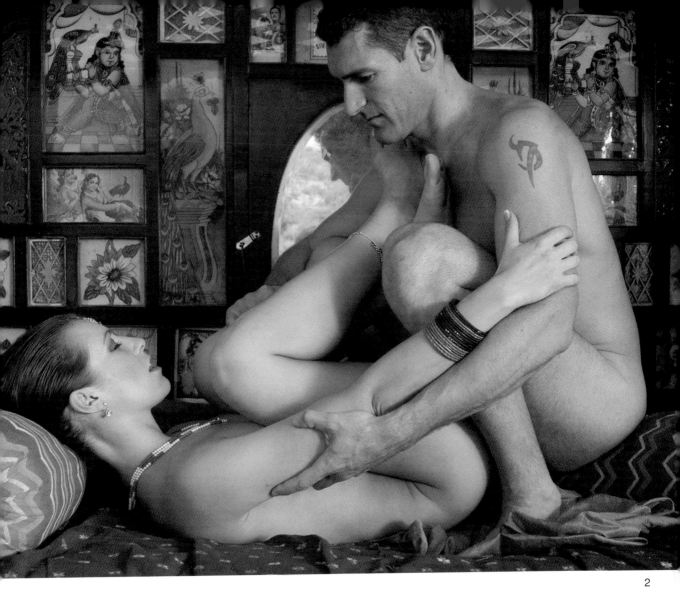

2

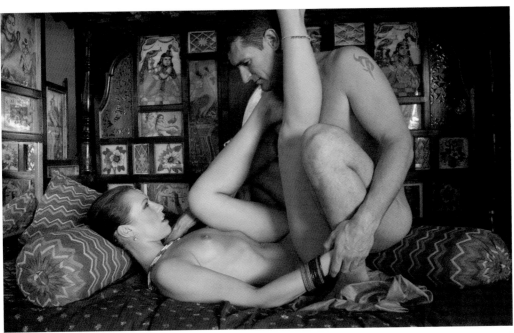

3

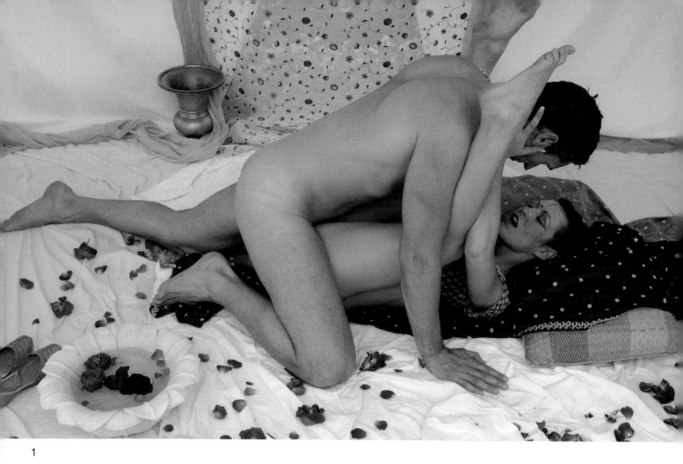

1

The "spoons position" is a beautifully tender embrace to move into when your lovemaking is winding down. Bodies pressed against each other, you can relax and drift into sleep feeling loved and protected.

3 spoons

2

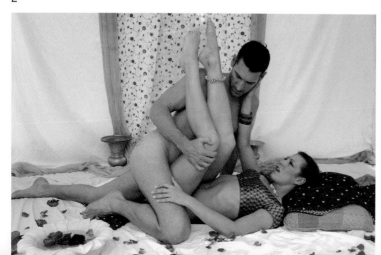

This peaceful sequence starts with a deeply penetrative position and subsides gently into "spoons." At the height of passion, a position that allows deep penetration is extremely satisfying. With both lovers fully aroused, the "alternate yawning position" is an erotic variation on the missionary position. The woman lies on her back and raises her legs high in the air. The man lies between her legs, resting his weight on his knees and hands, with his arms to the outside of his lover's thighs and arms (1).

The woman's calves can be on her partner's upper arms or, if they start to ache, she can bend her knees around his elbows. The man uses rhythmic thrusting movements, easily controlling the speed, depth, and angle of penetration, and his lover can also aid his movements by holding and moving his hips.

As the intensity of your passion starts to ease, the woman brings down her left leg and lifts her right leg over her partner to meet it (2). The man rolls onto his right side, as his lover moves her body at right angles to his and places both her legs over his thighs (3). The man rests his head on his right arm, and the woman raises her right arm to hold his head, as the lovers gaze into each other's eyes. After the vigorous passion of the previous position, the side-by-side "carriage" is a perfect resting posture.

Now, to nestle together "spoons-style," the woman brings both legs over her partner's, turns onto her left side and moves her body around so that her back is pressed against her lover's chest (4). He can nuzzle his face into the back of her neck and clasp her waist or caress her breasts with his right hand. Try

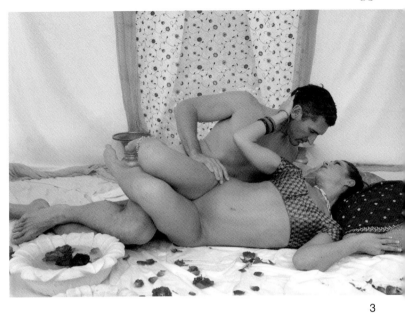

3

breathing in tune with each other, sustaining the connection between you, as you drift peacefully off in your own world.

4

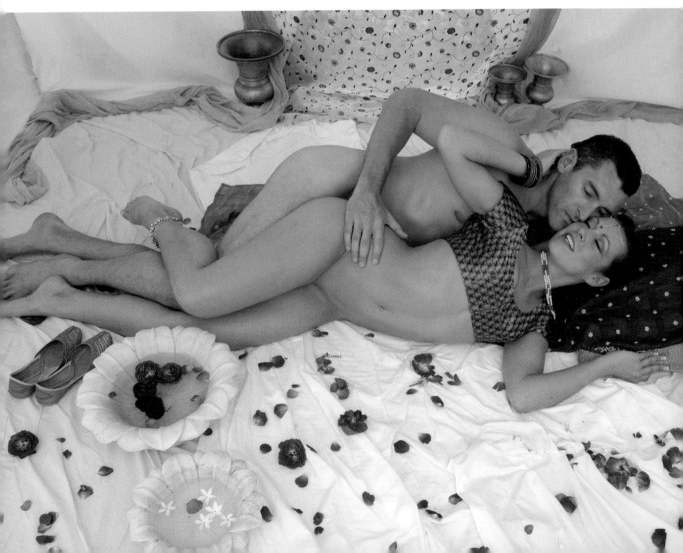

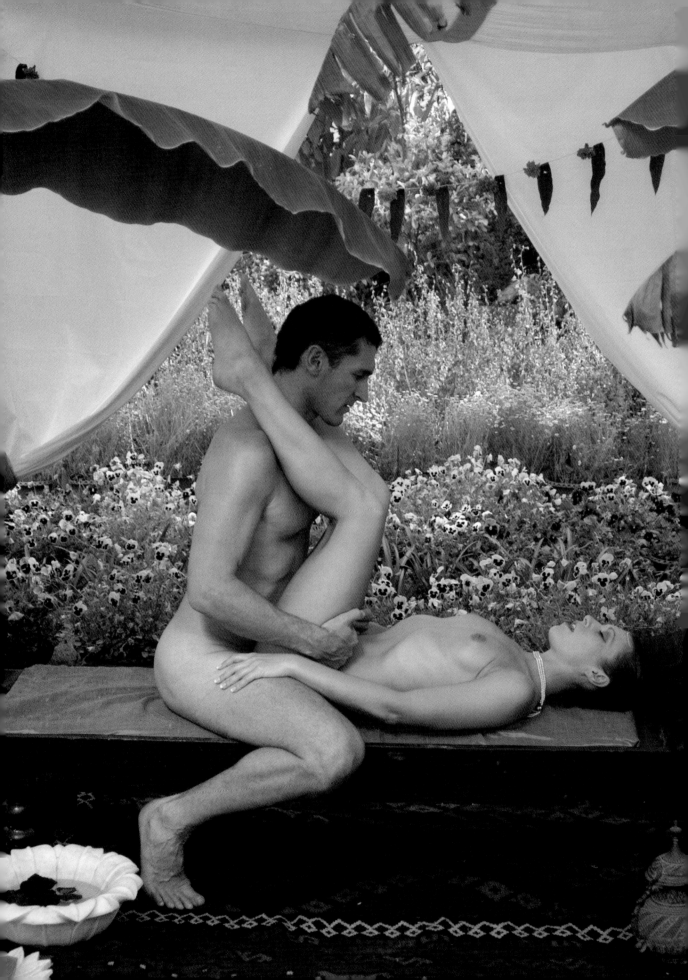

IN THE GARDEN *Props, such as garden furniture, provide a useful support when trying out different lovemaking positions. Make sure it is sturdy, and cover it with soft fabrics and pillows for extra comfort.*

4 sky foot

"Sky foot" makes great use of a garden table for easy access. The woman lies on the edge of the table, holding onto the sides, while the man stands or sits between her legs. She reclines, he moves forward and, as he enters her, she raises her legs straight up so that her thighs rest on his stomach (main picture).

From this position he can alternate deep and shallow thrusts and, by pushing her hands down on the table, the woman can lift her hips and move them in a delicious circling motion. She can also bring her legs together and slightly cross them to alter the pleasurable sensations against the wall of her yoni.

When the excitement becomes too intense, the "fixing a nail" position offers a gentle interlude. The woman raises one leg and places the heel of her foot on her lover's forehead. He caresses her foot (2), they rest for a few moments, and then she brings that leg down to his shoulder and stretches out the other (3). Slowly repeating this—raising and extending each leg alternately—is called "splitting the bamboo" and has the effect of massaging the lingam in an exquisite fashion.

RHYTHMS OF LOVE

Part of the beauty of nature lies in its rhythms—the changing seasons, the ebb and flow of the tides, the waxing and waning moon. As a passionate dance between lovers, great sex also has its own varying cadences. Incorporating the rhythms of nature into your lovemaking can be sensational.

In tidal lore, the seventh wave of the sea is always the strongest: for a teasing rhythm based on the swell of the ocean, try six shallow thrusts of the lingam followed by a seventh deep one and repeat.

Varying the style, pace, and number of thrusting rhythms also helps prolong lovemaking, as the level of stimulation never becomes overwhelming. Hip circling— either partner turning their hips in half-circles, first one way then the other—can also be highly arousing.

2

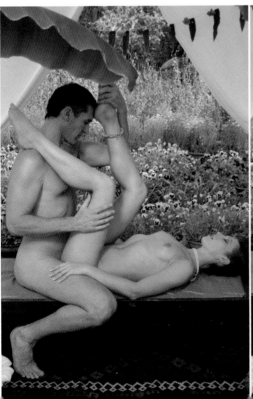

3

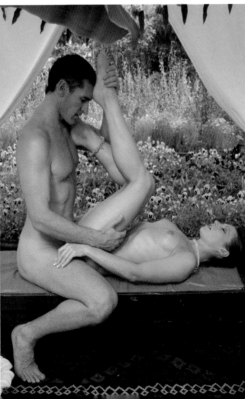

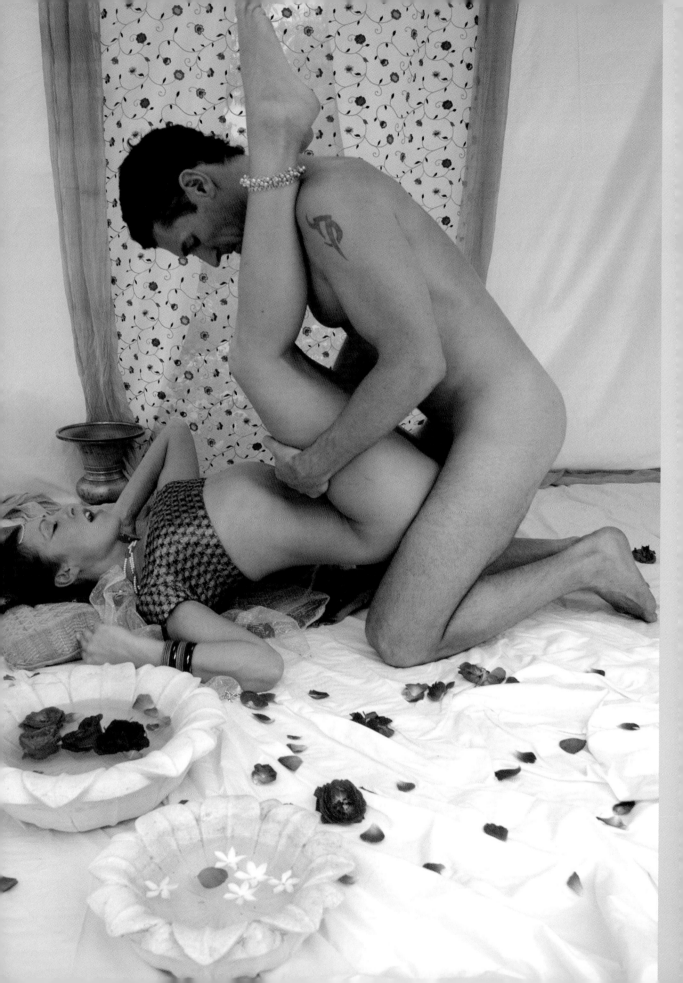

The "arrow of love" is a beautiful position to try on your garden bench or a low couch. Make sure you have plenty of soft pillows for the woman to lie on and to ease the pressure on the man's knees.

5 arrow of love

The woman reclines and raises her legs up so that her thighs rest against the sides of her breasts, holding them back with her hands. As her lover enters her she arches her body in the shape of a bow and rests her ankles on his shoulders as he holds her thighs (main picture), or passes his arms under her legs while supporting his weight with his hands on the couch, or reaches behind her to grip the top of the back of the bench. With the opening of her yoni receiving strong stimulation in this position, her lover can alter his position (1) and vary the depth and style of his thrusts.

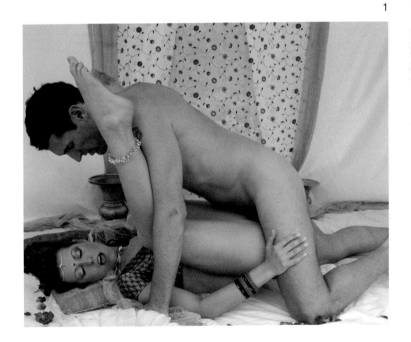

1

MOVEMENTS OF LOVE

The Kama Sutra offers some exciting variations on the "movements of love" that you can try. Vatsyayana suggests:

- Moving forward—when the organs are brought together properly and directly
- Churning—when the lingam is held with the hand and turned all around in the yoni
- Piercing—when the yoni is lowered, and the upper part of it is struck with the lingam
- Rubbing—when the same thing is done with the lower part of the yoni
- Pressing—when the yoni is pressed by the lingam for a long time
- Giving a blow—when the lingam is removed to some distance from the yoni, and then forcibly strikes it
- Blow of a boar—when one part of the yoni is rubbed with the lingam
- Blow of a bull—when both sides of the yoni are rubbed this way
- Sporting of a sparrow—when the lingam is in the yoni, and moved up and down frequently, and without being taken out

HITTING THE MARK

"With the woman's body now bent into the shape of a bow, he should aim his 'arrow of love.' This is a particularly fine lovemaking position which is much enjoyed by both partners."

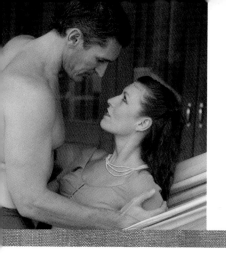

The following exciting sequence of positions uses the natural swinging movement of the hammock to enhance the erotic sensations you experience in this classic Kama Sutra pose.

6 wife of Indra

If you are lucky enough to have a hammock in your yard, make the most of it! A double-sized hammock (covered with a soft blanket for extra comfort, if it is made of string) and a good sense of balance are recommended for the "wife of Indra" sequence.

The woman reclines sideways in the hammock, her legs apart and swinging over the edge. The man stands in front of her between her legs and, holding her hands, lifts her up to a sitting position (1). As he does this, she raises her legs up so that her buttocks and the heels of her feet are resting on the very edge of the hammock, and her thighs are drawn up close to her body.

The man grips the hammock and gently swings her on to his erect lingam, in the "wife of Indra" position (2). She holds his lingam tightly in her yoni and uses the swinging of the hammock to slide along his lingam with sensational results. The woman can hold her lover's hips to control the movement, or steady the edge of the hammock with her hands (3).

As her legs start to tire, the woman stretches them out along the sides of her lover's waist and then bends her knees and places her feet on his hips. Now she can push herself on and off him as he holds her hips or feet, swinging her slowly backward and forward. Finally, she perches on the edge of the hammock and wraps her legs around her lover for a close embrace.

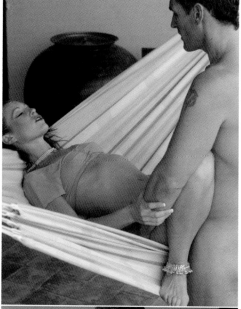

1

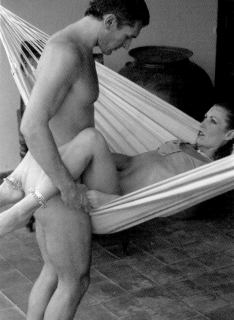

2

In The Garden

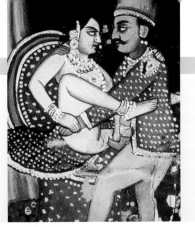

This playful miniature shows just how inventive the lovers of ancient India could be with their use of props in lovemaking.

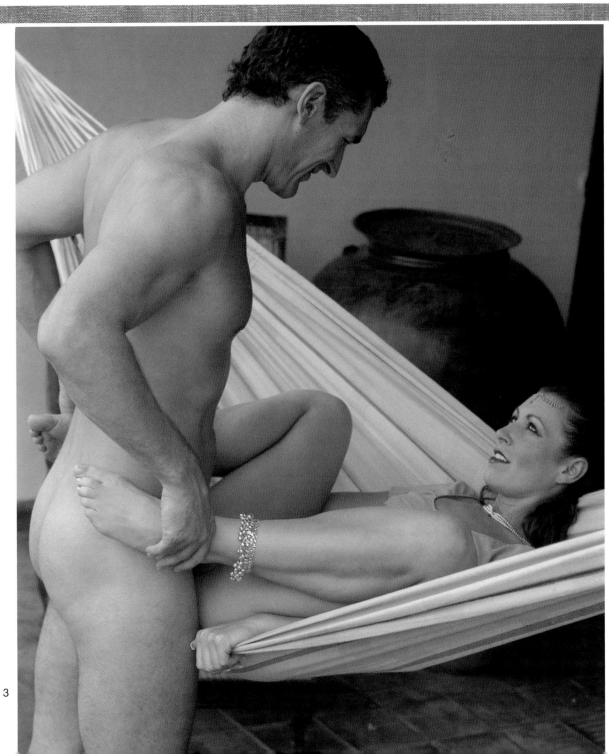

PLAYFUL POSITIONS *Playful sex means letting your imagination run wild, trying new things, and not caring how silly you look! It embodies the spirit of carefree lovemaking that happens naturally at the beginning of a relationship.*

7 *the* monkey

The "monkey" sequence is a seated position in which the woman is lifted up by her lover and moved around on his lingam before she turns in his lap, while still united, to face away from him. It's not easy but it's a fun position to play around with, especially if you feel moved to mimic the noises of the animal you're imitating.

The man kneels with the woman sitting astride him on his lap. He raises her up, by passing his arms under her legs, and uses his elbows to move her backward and forward, toward and away from him. The woman supports herself with her arms outstretched behind her, hands on the ground (1).

The "monkey" becomes the "roaring position" if the man uses his elbows to move his lover from side to side. Feel free to add your own "roaring" sound effects!

This position can be tiring for the man unless he has very strong arm muscles; he can rest between movements by kneeling forward slightly and gently placing his lover down onto a pillow while still staying within her.

To reverse the monkey, the woman lifts her left leg (2) and passes it over the head of her lover. She is now sitting on his lap "sidesaddle" (3), a lovely position for close, cradling embracing. She gently turns her body so that she is facing away from her partner (4).

IMAGINATIVE SEX

"An ingenious person should multiply the kinds of congress after the fashion of the different kinds of beasts and of birds. For these different kinds of congress, performed according to the usage of each country, and the liking of each individual, generate love, friendship, and respect in the hearts of women."

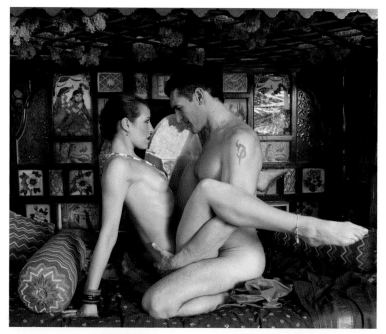

1

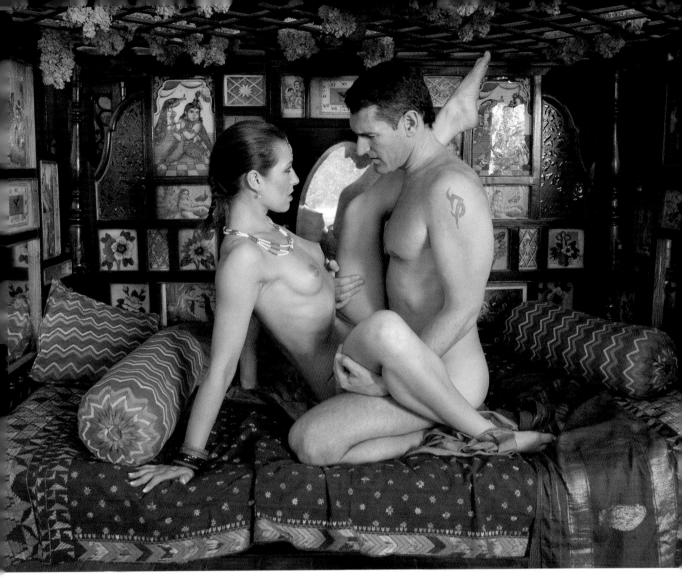

2

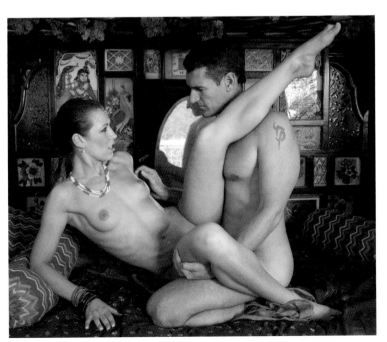

3

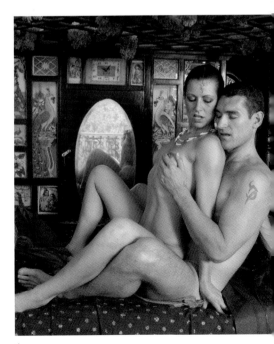

4

It is exciting to move from one position to another while keeping the lingam and yoni united. Here is a way of reversing direction—without withdrawing—that can be attempted in a spirit of playfulness.

8 turning position

The man lies on top of the woman with his legs between hers (1). He carefully raises his left leg and then his right over her right leg. Using his arms as support, and without withdrawing, he slowly moves both legs around (2).

Finally, he is facing in the opposite direction with his thighs either side of his lover's waist. The woman can now grip his waist with her thighs as he thrusts back into her (3). You can also kiss each other's feet (4).

Sex is a celebration of joy and openness, and being able to laugh and play together is part of the process of building trust and intimacy. Much of the fun of trying challenging positions is when you collapse in a heap of giggles together, and then kiss and try something new.

Having sex outdoors adds a playful edge from the start of your lovemaking, and seeking inspiration from the mating habits of the animal kingdom, as Vatsyayana suggests in the Kama Sutra, can help kick-start your imagination to come up with your own fresh and exciting positions.

1

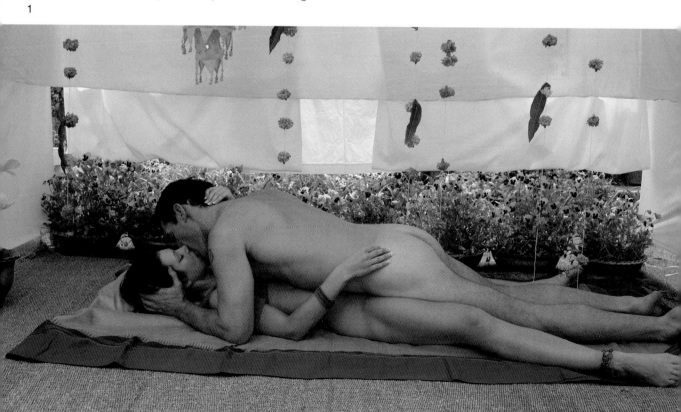

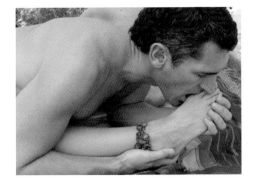

2

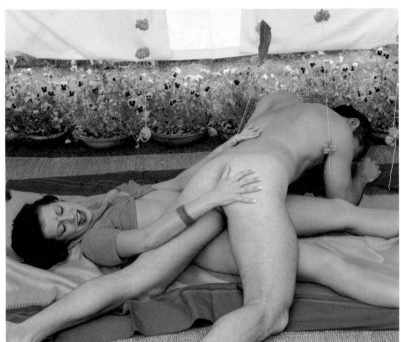

4

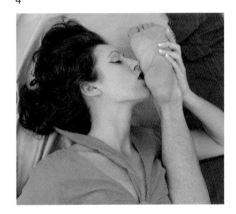

*The foot was an erotic
part of the body in India
and kissing your lover's
feet is an act of pure
tenderness.*

3

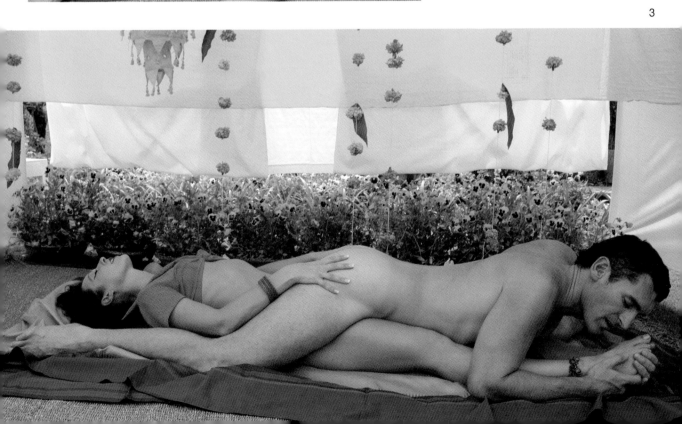

As well as enabling deep penetration, rear-entry positions are visually exciting for the man and also allow him to reach around and caress his lover's breasts and provide extra clitoral stimulation.

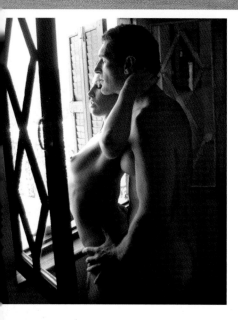

1

9 *the* zookeeper

The following sequence begins with one of the more challenging standing postures. Using a tree or window sill as a support, the woman stands with her back to the man and leans back against him. He caresses her stomach, hips (1), and breasts and reaches down around the front of her thigh to stroke her clitoris.

When the lovers can hold back no longer, he bends his knees and enters her from behind, in the "ass" position (main picture). Clasping her hips and waist, he can move her up and down on his lingam as she bends and straightens her legs, rising up to her toes if need be, depending on the difference in heights.

This is a strenuous position; as the man's legs begin to tire, the woman bends forward from the waist and, reaching down to the ground with her hands (or resting them on a pillow or tree trunk), moves into "congress of a cow." The man can grip her hips for stronger thrusting, and bends forward from the waist to cover her back with his body in a clasping embrace.

Still united, the lovers gently lower themselves to the ground and, as the man kneels behind the woman, continue in the "elephant position." Here, the woman kneels, rests on her elbows with her head raised, and can help direct the speed and depth of the man's movements with her own hip movements. She can also use a churning motion, rise up higher onto her hands or sink further into the ground with hips raised as the passion increases.

IMAGINATIVE SEX

"When a woman stands on her hands and feet like a quadruped, and her lover mounts her like a bull, it is called the 'congress of a cow.' At this time everything that is ordinarily done on the bosom should be done on the back. In the same way can be carried on the congress of a dog, the congress of a goat, the congress of a deer, the forcible mounting of an ass, the congress of a cat, the jump of a tiger, the pressing of an elephant, the rubbing of a boar, and the mounting of a horse. And in all these cases the characteristics of these different animals should be manifested by acting like them."

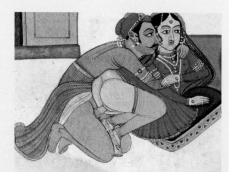

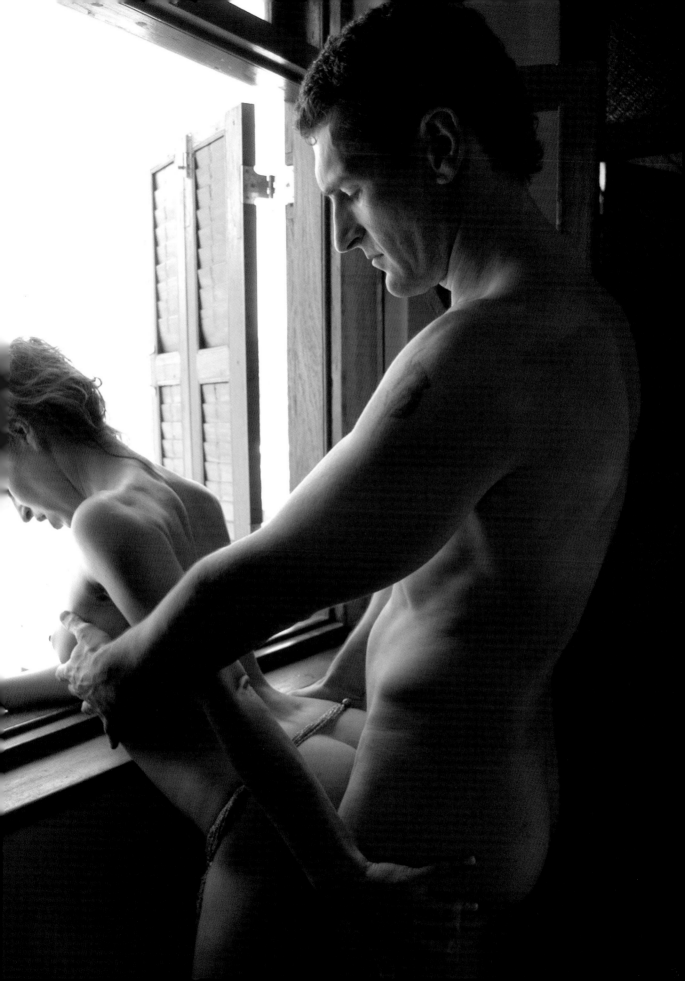

SPONTANEOUS POSITIONS *Standing positions are perfect for spontaneous lovemaking when you are overcome by desire. The Kama Sutra suggests using a "wall or pillar" for "supported congress." In a natural setting, a tree is ideal.*

10 climbing of a tree

This beautifully tender standing embrace is another that can easily be adopted when overcome by passion and in a hurry. Again, a tree offers good support. This sequence starts with the "knee elbow" position. This position works best if the woman is much lighter than her lover; if this isn't the case, be careful to avoid back strain and, if need be, move straight to the "climbing of a tree."

The man rests his weight against a tree and, keeping his knees slightly bent, takes his lover in his arms. As they unite, she "climbs" up him, with her arms around his shoulders, until her feet are toward the middle of his thighs and her bent knees are level with his elbows. Her lover supports her knees with his elbows and uses his hands to give extra support to her legs (main picture). If his arms are strong he will be able to lift her up and down. The "knee elbow" is a deeply passionate position but it is one that requires much strength in the man.

As the woman drops one leg down and places her foot on the foot of her lover, he supports her other foot in the palm of his hand—a very tender gesture. She embraces him with one arm around his back and the other on his shoulders and then rests her raised foot on his thigh, in the "climbing of a tree" position.

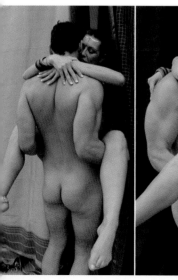 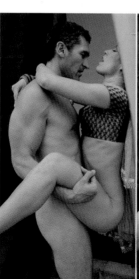 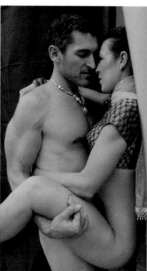 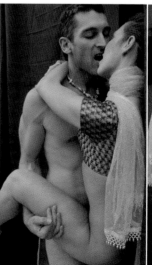 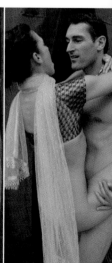

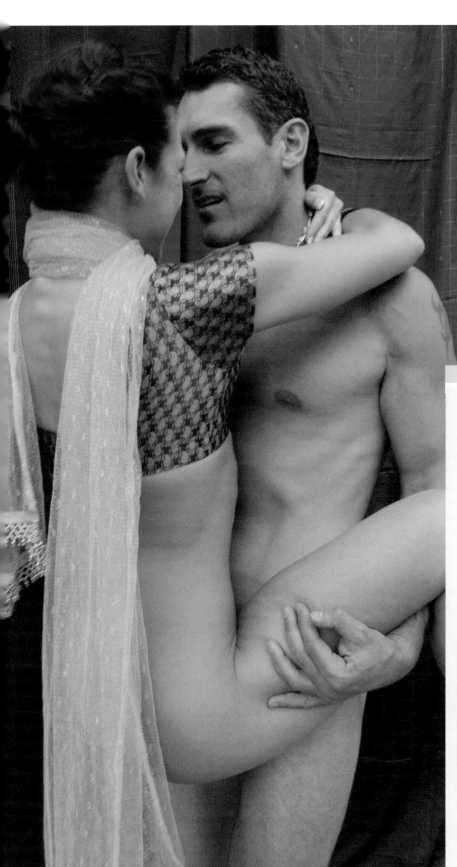

TENDER EMBRACE

"When a woman, having placed one of her feet on the foot of her lover, and the other on one of his thighs, passes one of her arms around his back, and the other on his shoulders, makes slightly the sounds of singing and cooing, and wishes, as it were, to climb up him in order to have a kiss, it is called an embrace like the 'climbing of a tree.'"

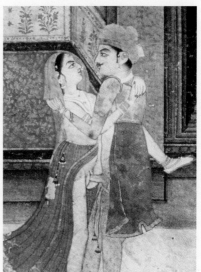

"When a woman, clinging to a man as a creeper twines around a tree, bends his head down to hers with the desire of kissing him and slightly makes the sound of sut sut, embraces him, and looks lovingly toward him, it is called an embrace like the 'twining of a creeper.'"

twining of a creeper

Walking through the woods hand-in-hand with your lover, you reach a secluded glade or clearing with dappled sunlight shining in soft rays through the branches of the trees. You stop, embrace, and start to kiss. Carried away by desire, you rest against a tree and let your passion take its course.

The man leans back against the tree and his lover embraces him (1). The woman raises one leg and wraps it around the outside of her lover's thigh in order for him to enter her while he supports her by holding her waist and buttocks. With the man standing firm, like a tree, and the woman with one foot on the ground, the lover's are in the "tripod position." They have three feet on the ground while the man supports his partner's raised leg by holding her thigh (main picture). Twining her body around her lover, the woman wraps her raised leg around her lover's leg and embraces him passionately (2). The man's movements are limited in this position—especially if the bark of the tree is rough against his back—so it is up to the woman to control the depth and pace of lovemaking, although her lover can help her by supporting some of her weight and she may also be able to brace herself against tree branches.

TAKING CARE

The standing positions require a strong back in the man and flexibility in the woman. Take care not to overdo it in the heat of passion. Always bend from your knees when lifting your partner and keep your movements slow and smooth. If you have back problems, avoid lifting and carrying your lover.

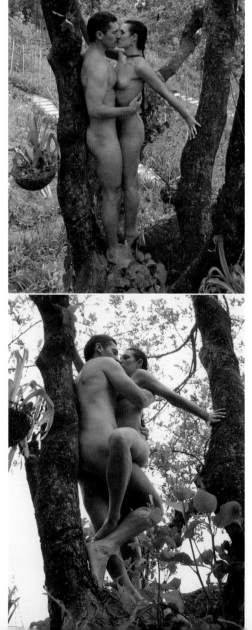

1

2

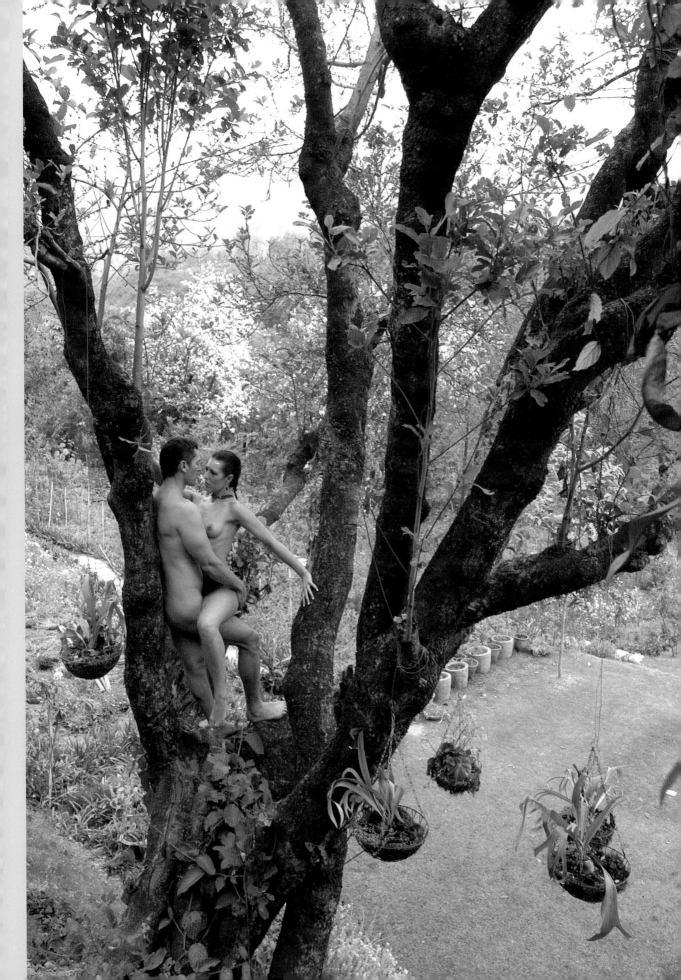

Positions that do not require you to remove too many clothes or much movement are ideal for spontaneous sex, especially when you're not totally sure the spot you've chosen is completely secluded.

12 *the* pair of tongs

This position relies on the woman having strong vaginal muscles. The man sits on the ground, perhaps resting against a tree or log. The woman sits in his lap, his lingam inside her. Using her "love muscle," she grips his lingam and uses a steady squeeze-and-release technique, or a fluttering motion like a butterfly's wings.

In this position, penetration is deep but all the movement is within the woman's yoni so, with careful layering of clothes or a blanket, it looks like you are just enjoying a close embrace.

THE LOVE MUSCLE

For women, "pair of tongs" is an ideal position in which to make use of your pelvic floor, or "love muscle." This is the muscle you use to stop the flow of urine. To locate it, place a finger inside your vagina, and feel the pulling and squeezing sensation as you grip and relax.

For an invisible love-muscle workout that can be done anywhere, draw up your pelvic floor muscles, hold for 10 seconds then relax and repeat, up to 10 times. You can also try quickly tightening and releasing for 10 repetitions. Build up the number of repetitions gradually.

Playing with this muscle during sex becomes an art form as you discover how to grip, ripple, fan, caress, and massage your lover's lingam without appearing to move an inch! Most women find that a toned love muscle enhances arousal during sex, and creates stronger orgasms, while men enjoy the firmer gripping sensation. In any position, try a brief squeeze as the lingam is withdrawn during a shallow thrust, and a longer squeeze that lasts the duration of a deeper thrust. Another pleasurable technique is to squeeze slowly as your partner slowly enters or withdraws.

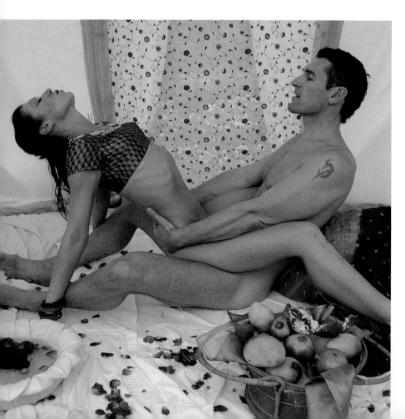

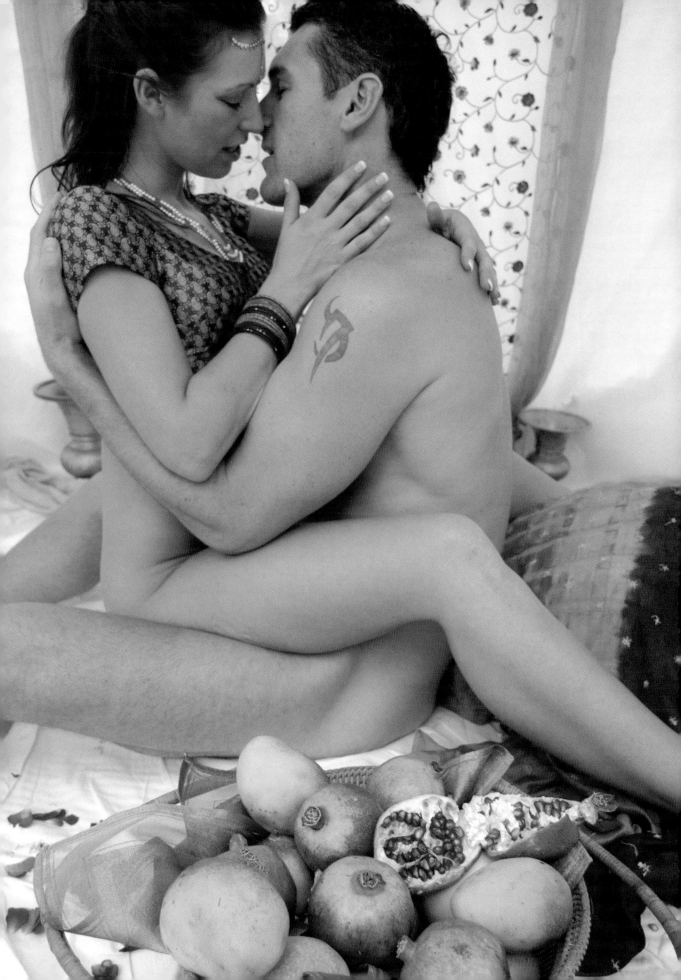

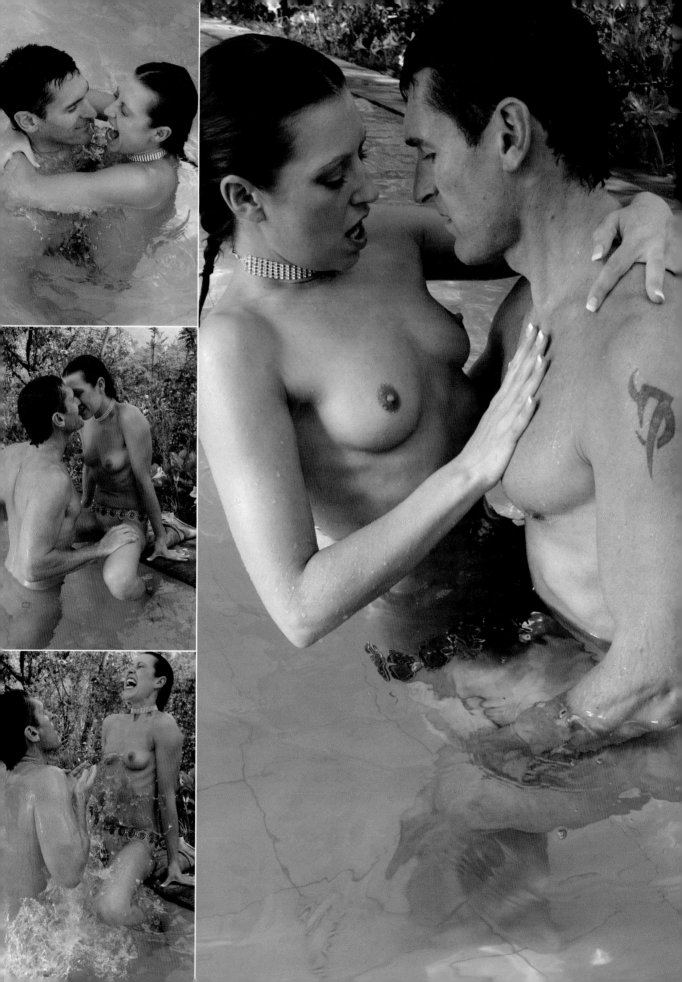

IN THE WATER *Splashing about in water is a sensual experience that lends itself perfectly to lovemaking, whether you are on a beach, in a private swimming-pool, by the shores of a lake, or playing in a stream.*

the mermaid

13

Aquatic sex is great for standing postures as the water supports your weight, making it easier to experiment. You can brace yourselves against the sides of the pool for extra support, or, in the sea, you might be able to find a suitable rock.

After playing in the water, kissing, splashing, and enjoying the feel of the warm water all over your bodies (far left), embrace closely, enjoying the sensation of your wet bodies touching. If you feel confident about holding your breath under water, you could go under the water and tease each other orally. Come up for breath before you feel you really need to, then take another full breath and go down again. If you're being pleasured in this way, be careful not to hold your lover's head under the water in your excitement.

When you are both fully aroused, the woman clasps her lover around the neck and wraps her legs around his waist (main picture). He enters her. Up-and-down movement is easy with the help of the water (below). Keep your balance by taking little steps forward or backward every so often and by moving your arms in the water. Enjoy tumbling over together into the water as you climax!

SAFE SEX IN WATER

Sex in water is a fantastic experience but there are some basic precautions to take to make it safe and pleasurable. Condoms can easily slip off in water so avoid full intercourse if you are practicing safer sex or using condoms as your only means of contraception. Water can also wash away natural lubricants, so placing a little artificial lubricant in your vagina beforehand makes penetration more comfortable. Be careful of currents, however slow-moving, in rivers, streams, and the sea. Take care not to get so involved in your fun that you drift beyond your safe swimming distance.

If you decide to take your water fun indoors to the shower, always stand on a non-slip rubber mat.

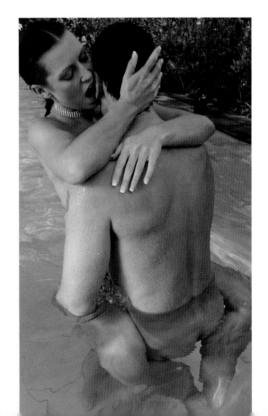

"Sporting of swans" is a woman-on-top sequence—pure delight for the man. It is a lovely position to try on the shoreline with gentle waves lapping against your bodies.

14 sporting of swans

The man lies down comfortably on his back. His lover lowers herself onto him and squats above him. If comfortable, she can place her feet on his hips. This is the traditional posture—the woman may need to steady herself by clasping her lover's raised hands, and should be careful to place her heels directly on the man's hips. Alternatively, she can place her feet on the ground on either side of his buttocks (1).

As well as being an exciting position for the man, this is extremely satisfying one for the woman as she can control the angle of penetration and the speed of thrusting—she moves up and down, or circles her pelvis— and her lover can reach up to caress her. From this posture, known as the "bee buzzing over man" position (see panel), the woman places one foot on her lover's chest and then brings it around to meet her other foot so that she has both feet on one side of her lover (2) and supports herself on her elbows or hands on his other side. This is the "sporting of swans" position (3).

1

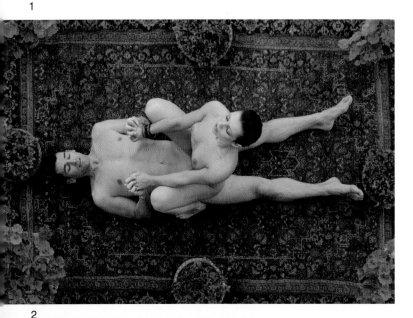

2

TAKING PLEASURE

"The wife, having placed her husband at full length, sits at squat upon his thighs, closes her legs firmly after she has effected insertion; and, moving her waist in a circular form, churning as it were, enjoys her husband and thoroughly satisfies herself."

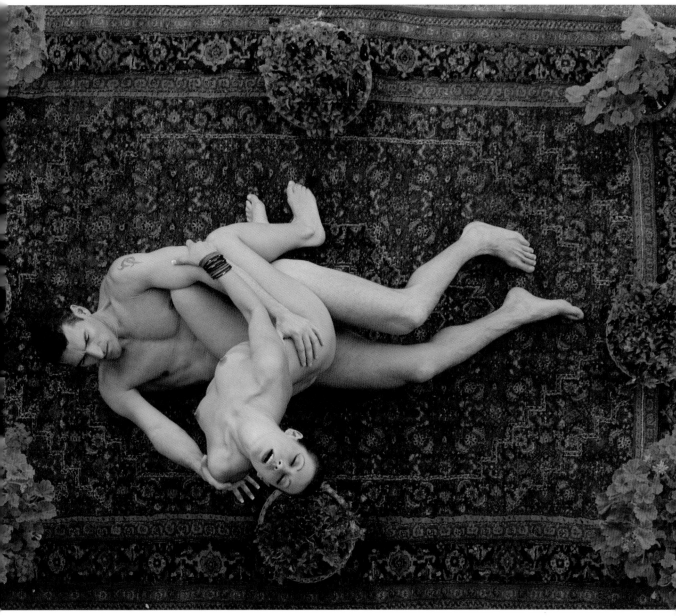

3

THE KALI POSTURE

The "bee buzzing over man" position is also known as the "Kali posture" after the fierce goddess Kali. She is honored as both "mother goddess"—the source of life—and also as a dark force of destruction. She is sometimes pictured squatting on the dead body of her consort, Shakti, which is where, unromantically, the posture takes its name.

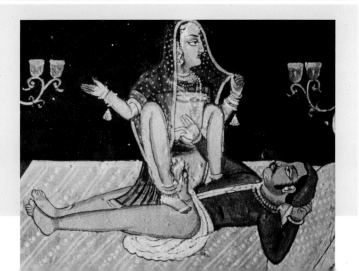

The final position in this sequence imitates the crab when it is moving, with its front claws drawn inward. It allows a great build-up of sexual tension in the woman's thighs and vaginal area.

15 *the* crab

The "crab" is another position that is fun to try on a beach, being tickled by the water, or on a sandbar adjoining a stream. Alternatively, this is a sensual position to try in your outdoor boudoir, where you can enjoy the softness of cushions for the woman to lie back on and to protect the man's knees.

The man kneels, comfortably sitting back on his heels. His lover sits astride him and clasps her hands around his neck. Lifting her feet off the ground (1), she leans back and raises her legs as the man supports her back with his hands (2). In this position you can rock gently backward and forward and the woman can deepen the angle of penetration by lifting her legs.

The woman now slowly lowers her back to the ground and raises both legs, bent at the knee, so that her thighs rest on her stomach (3). Her lover can continue to thrust from his kneeling position while caressing her legs.

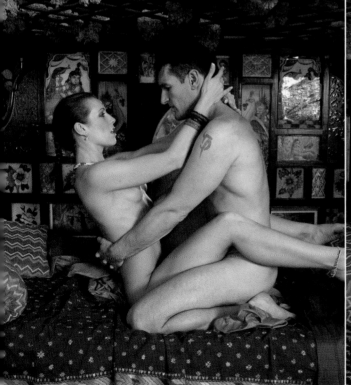

1

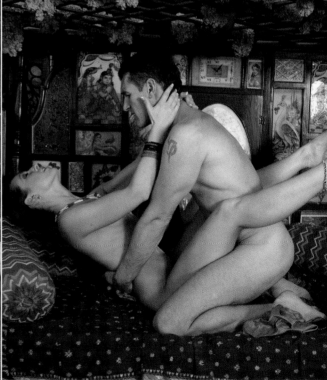

2

YOUR SACRED SPACE

To fully experience the delights of sex that incorporates mind, body, and soul, you need to allow yourselves a long stretch of time in a beautiful spot where there is no risk of being disturbed. Your outdoor boudoir of love is the ideal setting to explore this aspect of lovemaking. You can prepare your sacred space beforehand with everything you might need for a tantalizingly extended session of foreplay, including massage oils, treats to feed your lover, such as fresh fruit and squares of rich dark chocolate, and soft satin or velvet pillows to recline on. Allow yourselves to linger over pleasuring each other for as long as possible before uniting in penetrative sex.

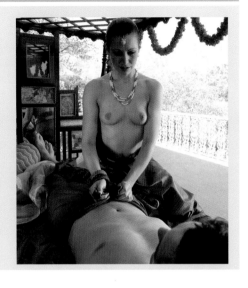

3

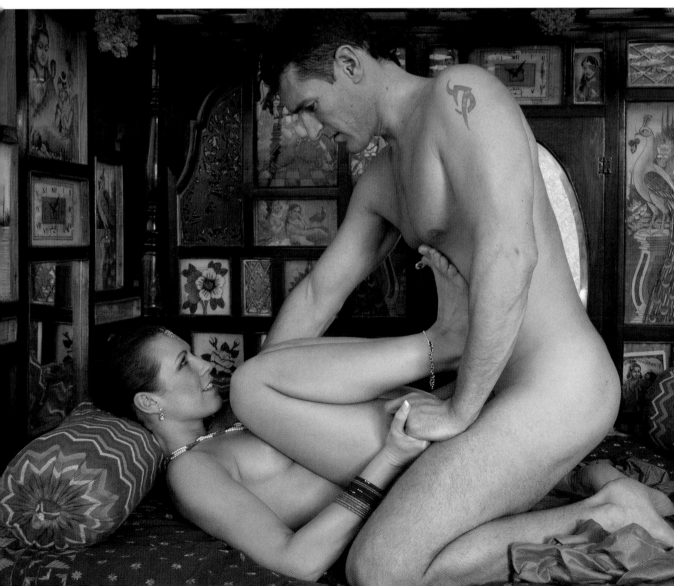

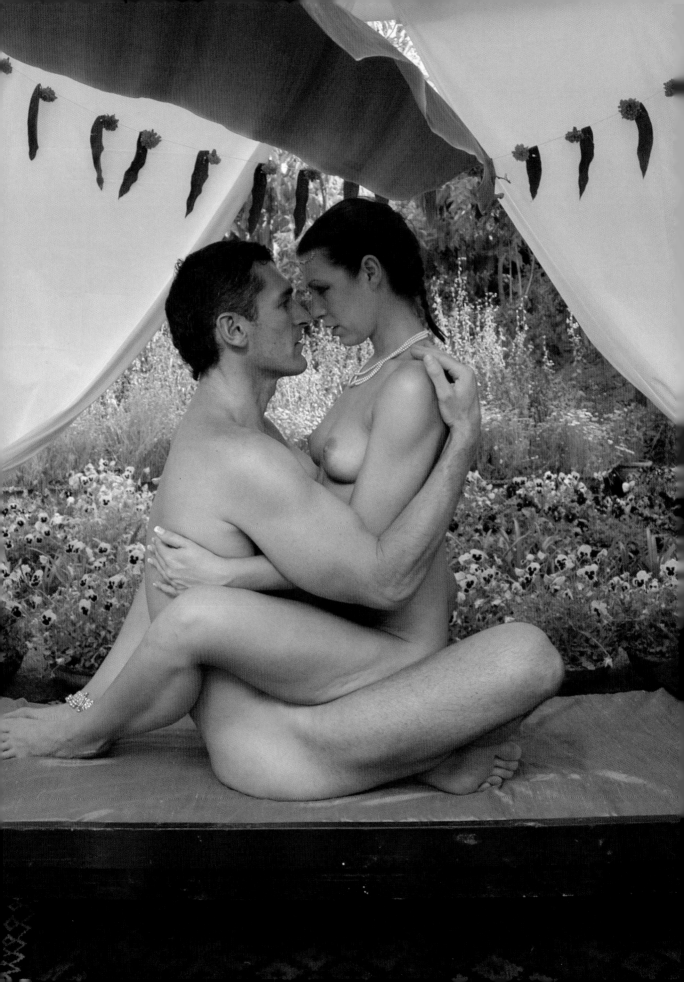

SPIRITUAL SEX *In the ancient Indian books of love, sex is more than just a profound expression of passion between lovers, it can also be a gateway to spiritual awakening and divine bliss.*

16 *the* lotus

In Tantric mythology the "lotus" position represents the union of the male and female principle and cosmic oneness. It is a loving, intimate embrace that creates a circuit of sexual energy between your two intertwined bodies.

The man sits in the lotus position (or with crossed legs if the lotus is too intense) and the woman sits on his lap and wraps her legs around his waist. They gaze into each other's eyes and feel the love connection between them (main picture). Then the woman gently lifts herself onto her lover's lingam.

While a limited amount of movement can be achieved in this intimate position by a gentle rocking of the pelvis (1) and by squeezing and relaxing the love muscle, the aim of the lotus is to become aware of the flow of sexual energy moving around your bodies.

Now place your arms, legs, and mouth so they exactly touch the corresponding parts of your partner's body. This is the "tortoise position," which creates an even stronger circuit of energy between your two bodies, especially if you complete it with deep, erotic kissing (2).

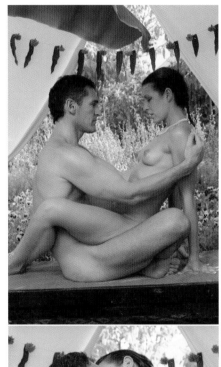

1

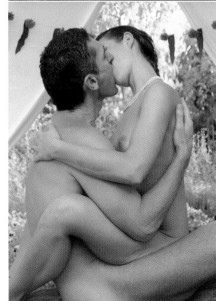

2

DIVINE ENERGY

In spiritual sex, you use the passion and power of erotic energy to explore the connection between body, mind, and spirit; when you surrender fully to each other in lovemaking you connect with the source of the universe itself. In the ancient Indian spiritual sex path called Tantra you enter the realm of the goddess. The creative force behind all existence is female, in the form of the goddess Shakti, and all women are honored as embodiments of the divine. According to Tantric wisdom, when Shakti unites with her god, Shiva, the entire world is created, in a sexual dance of bliss. Tantric couples honor each other as goddess and god, the divine male and female principles, and use lovemaking as a means to channel and transform sexual energy into spiritual awareness.

In divine sex, the harmonious shapes you make during lovemaking are designed to link the corresponding parts of your bodies and create circuits around which sexual energy can flow freely.

the snake trap

17

In the "snake trap," the man sits with his legs outstretched and the woman sits on his lap, her legs wrapped around his waist and in a strong embrace as you kiss and arouse each other (1). When the man's lingam is erect, the woman lifts herself on to it and stretches out her legs, then reaches behind her body to hold her lover's feet. The man holds onto both her feet (main picture).

There is no deep thrusting in this position, although you can both rock backward and forward to increase the level of stimulation. Enjoy the stillness of these intimate postures—try breathing in tune with each other, gaze into each other's souls, and discover the divine within your lover. The most important thing is that there's no need to rush. If the man loses his erection then simply change positions and engage in more foreplay before uniting again.

1

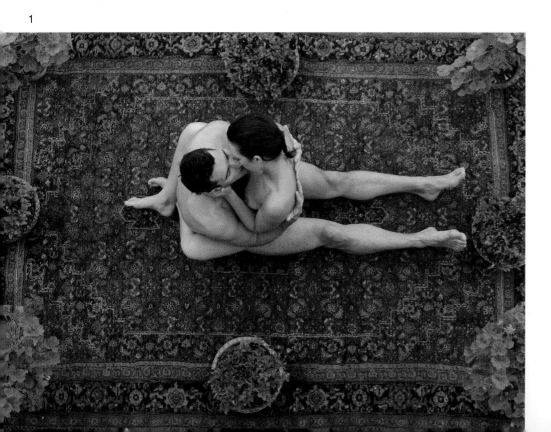

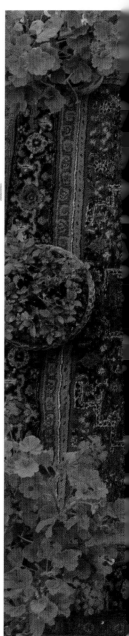

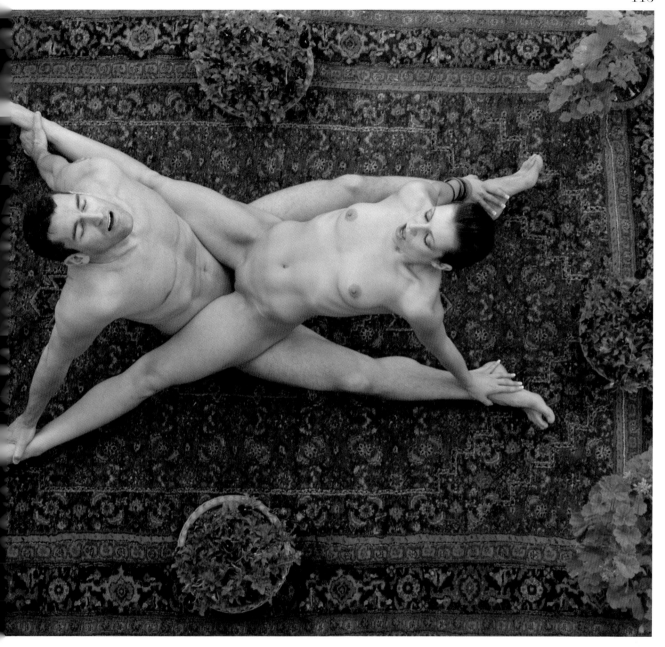

BREATH OF LIFE

Shared breathing is a very intimate form of non-verbal communication, nourishing your sense of connection with each other. Synchronize your breathing with your lover by inhaling and exhaling at the same time, in flow with the other.

Breathe in tune to create a peaceful rhythm to your lovemaking. Or create a circle of breathing—as you exhale, your lover inhales. This is described as the "binding breath" in some ancient Indian texts, as, with every breath, the lovers absorb the life-force of the other, and bestows their own. Breathe quickly with intensity for a "heating-up" effect that energizes and arouses. This is a good antidote to the tendency to hold the breath when reaching orgasm.

According to the ancient love manual, the Ananga-Ranga, the "wheel of kama" is a position "much enjoyed by voluptuous lovers." This gentle posture is considered to be a harmonious one in which to channel and resonate energy.

18 wheel of Kama

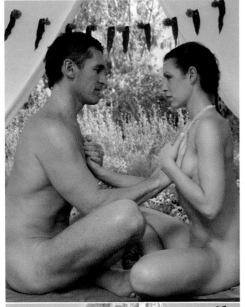

1

Sit opposite each other with legs crossed and knees touching. Each of you places your right palm on the other's heart. Now place your left hand over your lover's right hand, covering it (1). Gaze into each other's eyes and breathe in harmony, exhaling and inhaling at the same time. Feel the love connection between you, streaming out of your hearts and back in through your hands.

Keeping the same position, touch your foreheads together. Close your eyes and enjoy the feeling of closeness and intimacy (2). As you exhale, send your breath into your lover's third eye, in the center of the forehead. Pause while your lover inhales it from their third eye and exhales it back to you as you inhale.

Now, the man stretches out his legs and parts them. The woman sits on his lap, thighs gripping his waist and legs also outstretched. Hold each other's shoulders, lean backward and continue to soul gaze (3). When the time is right, the woman rises up and lowers herself onto her lover's lingam. At this point, reach for each other's hands and extend your arms out sideways (main picture) so that, from above, your outstretched arms and legs resemble the spokes of a wheel.

The woman can use her "love muscle" for vaginal fluttering in this position to maintain the erotic tension. As she tightens and releases her yoni around her lover's lingam, try to visualize the flow of sexual energy moving upward from your genitals and flowing through your bodies.

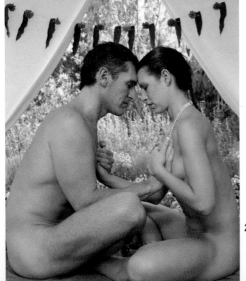

2

3

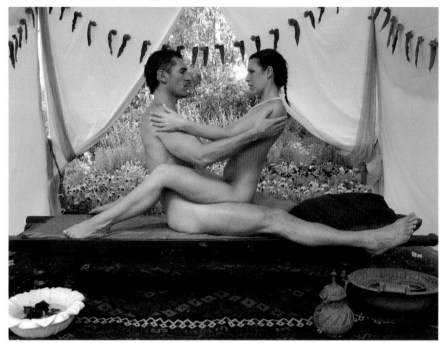

DELICIOUS HARMONY

*"How delicious an
instrument is woman,
when artfully played
upon; how capable is she
of producing the most
exquisite harmonies,
of executing the most
complicated variations of
love, and of giving the
most divine of erotic
pleasures."*
(Ananga-Ranga)

4

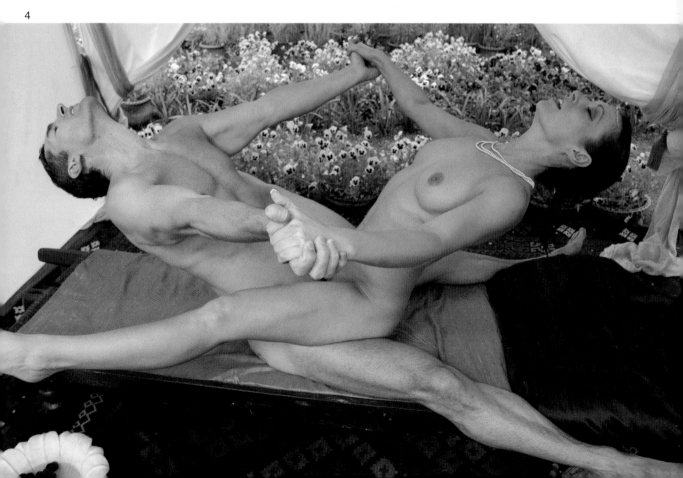

ADVENTUROUS POSITIONS *For more flexible couples, new and intense sensations may be experienced when you try adventurous positions that make the most of the suppleness of your bodies and imaginations.*

the swing

The *"swing"* is a woman-on-top position that offers delicious sensations for the woman and a novel view for the man. It can be adapted according to the suppleness of the man.

The man lies flat on his back with his lover straddling him, facing forward toward him and resting on her knees. With her heels hooked under his thighs and his hands clasping her waist or hips, she bends back into the *"cobra,"* her arms stretched out behind her and palms pressed down on the floor (1). As she leans back, she stretches out each leg in turn, so that her feet are on either side of her lover's head, and then gently lifts her left leg over his head to join her right leg (2). She carefully moves her body round (3)—supporting her weight on her hands by moving her left arm around the front of her body to meet her right arm—so that she is not twisting her lover's

1

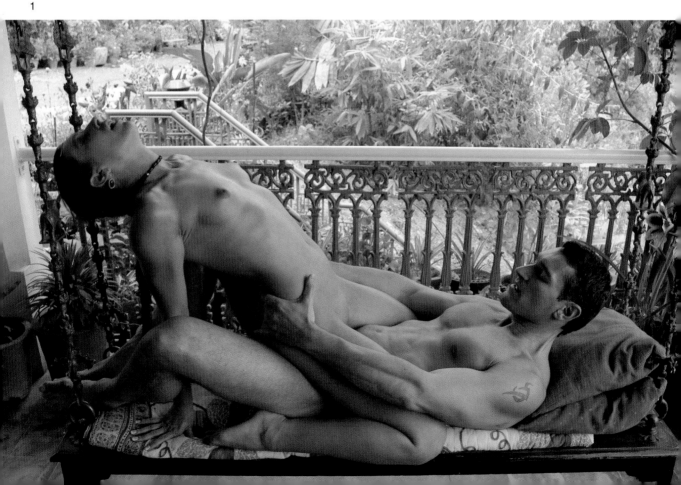

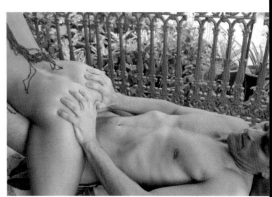

2

lingam, and ends up facing away from him (4).

In the traditional version, the man arches his back so that the middle part of his body is lifted off the ground while his lover, now raised up onto her feet, rocks backward and forward. If the man's back is not strong enough to do this then it is just as satisfying for him to be lying flat with the woman resting on her knees and either sitting up straight or resting forward on her hands. She can control the depth of penetration— perhaps teasing him by lifting up so that he is only slightly inside her and circling her hips then pushing down so that the whole length of him is inside—and he can caress her buttocks (5).

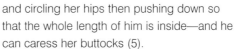

5

3

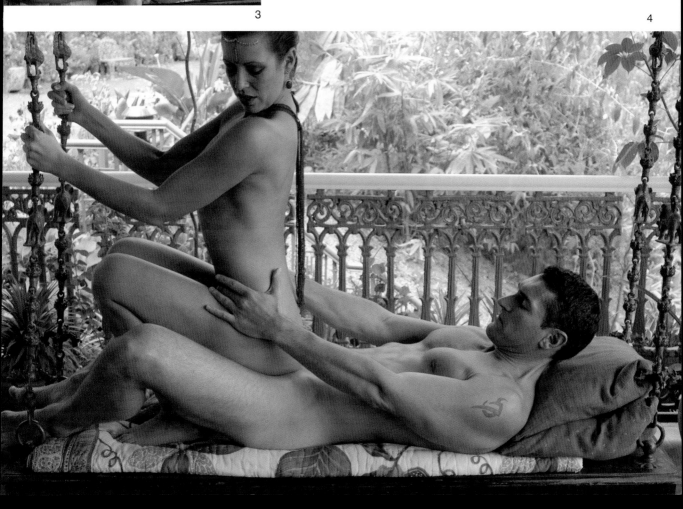

4

This exciting position requires the woman to have a supple back and strong arms. The reward is a pose that is both visually and physically stimulating.

the wheel

20

1

2

The woman lies on her back and draws up her legs so that the heels of her feet are close to her buttocks. She raises her arms and lifts them over her head, resting her hands on the ground with her fingers pointing toward her shoulders (1). She takes a deep breath then lifts her hips up off the ground, presses down through the palms of her hands and rests the crown of her head on the floor (2).

The man approaches, bends his knees and, holding her firmly, lifts her off the ground and enters her (main picture) as she supports herself with one foot still on the ground and the other leg wrapped around his body. The man firmly supports her weight with both hands and the woman wraps her other leg around his body, still supporting herself with her hands and crown on the ground.

You may not be able to hold this challenging position for very long but it benefits from an interesting angle of penetration for the man and, for the woman, making love with her head thrown back or upside down, can strongly intensify the sensations of orgasm.

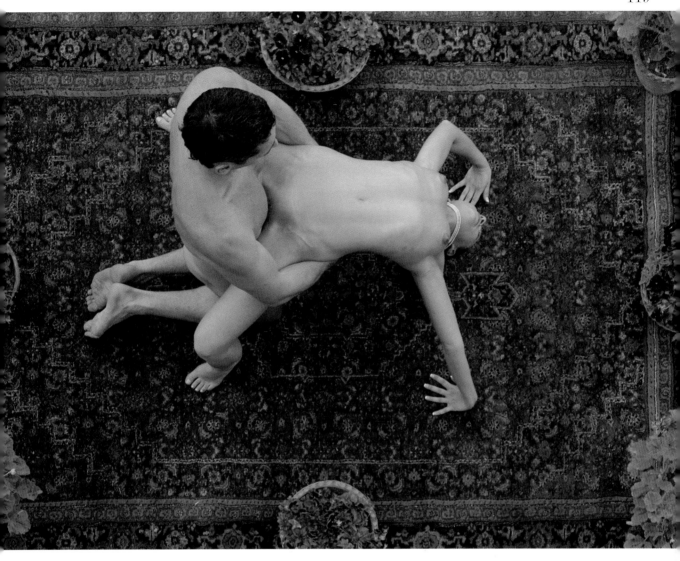

STRENGTH AND STAMINA

Some of the more adventurous positions require some strength, stamina, and flexibility. Couples in Vatsyayana's time would have honed these qualities in their bodies through the practice of yoga, and the same holds true today. Regular yoga work-outs can make a huge difference in strengthening and toning your body, opening up your hips and making your spine more flexible.

But yoga works on more than just the physical level. The Sanskrit word "yoga" means "to unite" or "yoke" and refers to the joining of body and mind. Yoga can help you feel more relaxed, so that you come to your lovemaking feeling centered, and better able to connect with your partner, and can open up your mind and body to deeper emotional feelings and sexual passion.

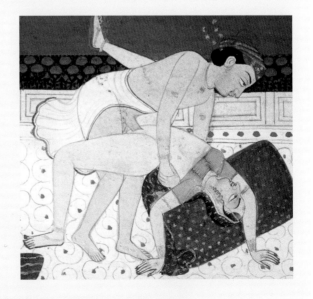

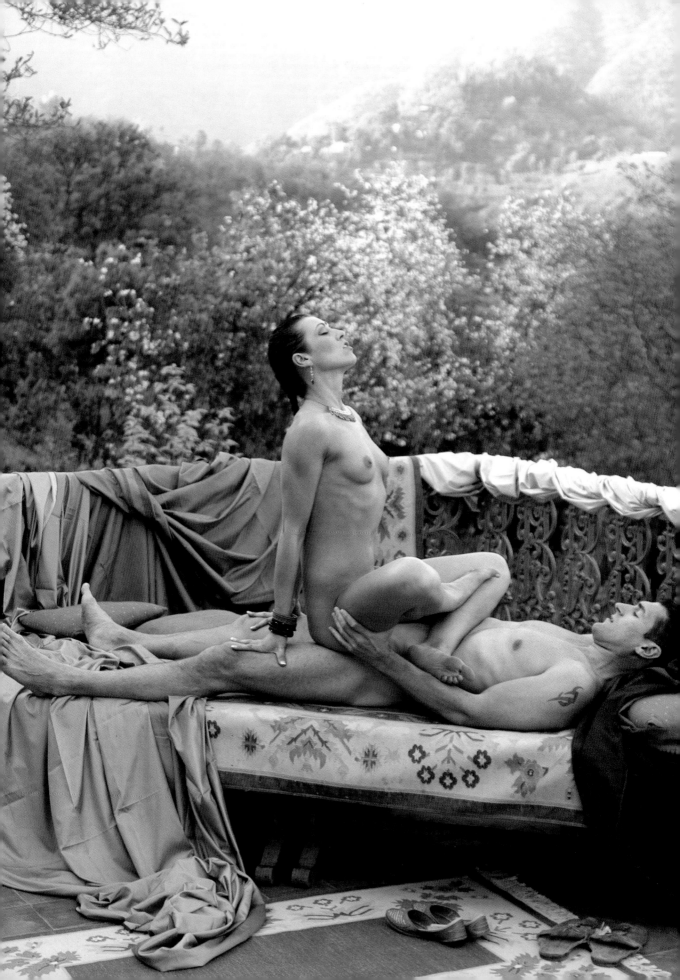

The "spinning top" is a classic Kama Sutra position. But it is also almost impossible and potentially dangerous for the man. This variation captures the spirit of the position— with less risk.

the spinning top

21

The man lies back with his legs straight. His lover straddles him with her knees bent and her feet on either side of his body. Using his knees as support, she leans back, raises her legs, and carefully crosses them so that she is in full lotus position, perched on her lover's lingam (main picture). From here she can rock herself forward and backward, sliding up and down the lingam in long, smooth strokes, rather than the circling of the classic *"spinning top."* If the man has strong arms he can also lift her up and down by placing his arms under her legs (2).

If the woman is unable to sustain the full lotus for very long she can rest her weight on each hand in turn on the ground as she uses the other hand to unfold each leg, place them on either side of her lover's body, so that her feet are by his head, and then press down on her hands to move her body (3).

2

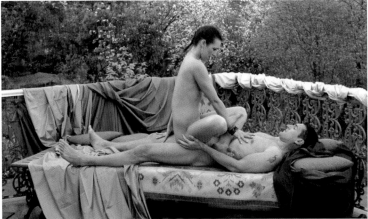

3

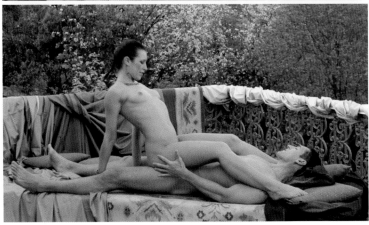

With her back arched and head thrown back in passion, the doves is a posture for the woman who has complete confidence in her own flexibility and in the strength of her lover.

22 *the* doves

This is an exciting and athletic position that requires a high level of flexibility in the woman and a strong back and arms in the man. The man sits on a chair and his lover sits on his lap facing him. He clasps his hands around her buttocks and gently pulls her onto him (1).

The woman begins to lean back, her legs now outstretched along either side of her lover's body, while he supports her back with his hands. She holds his arms to help her balance (2) and moves her hands down to his thighs as she continues to lower her body.

Finally, the woman leans back to her full extent, with her back arched and the crown of her head toward the floor. In this erotic pose, her lover grips her waist, supporting her lower back, and moves her gently (3).

This is a position that really emphasizes the level of trust between lovers. The woman needs to be able to relax into the pose, confident in the knowledge that her lover will support her physically and emotionally in this intense posture.

1

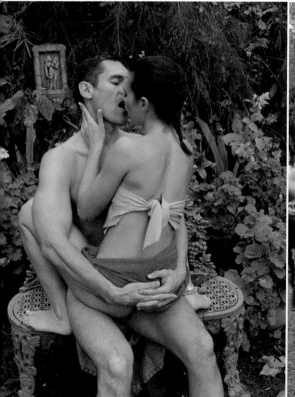

2

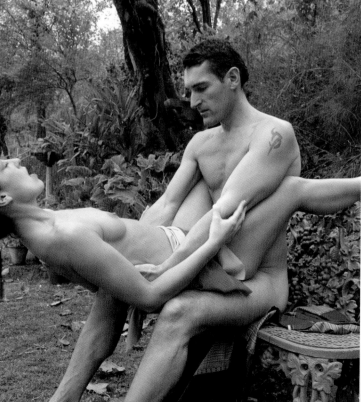

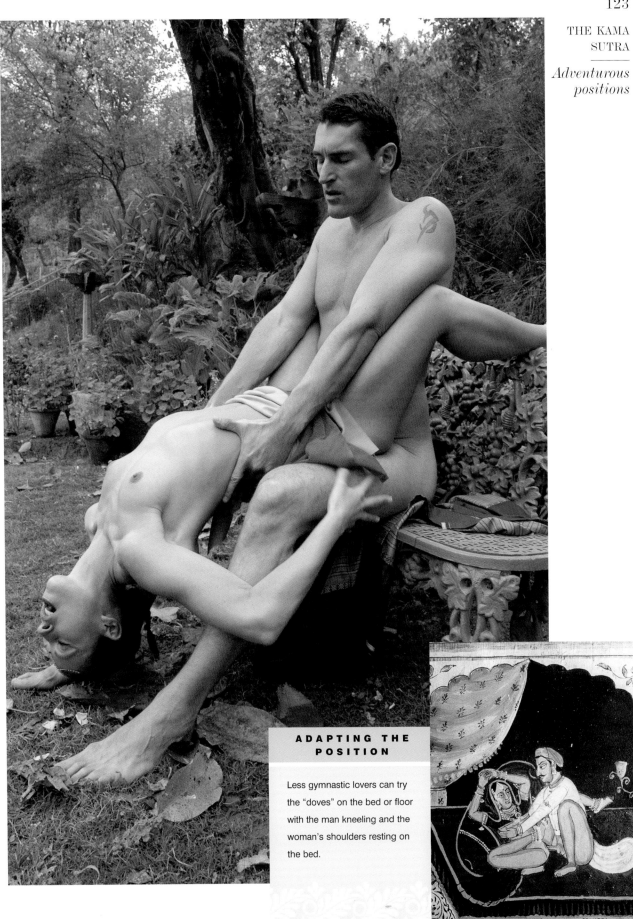

ADAPTING THE POSITION

Less gymnastic lovers can try the "doves" on the bed or floor with the man kneeling and the woman's shoulders resting on the bed.

Afterplay—enjoying the warm, blissful post-coital time of intimacy—is as vital to great lovemaking as foreplay. Just as lovemaking should start slowly, so it should also end slowly.

tender afterplay

When your lovemaking reaches its natural conclusion and you both lie happily exhausted in each other's arms, let the loving connection and mood you have nurtured continue for as long as possible. Try to stay in the moment and don't let your mind rush ahead to mundane thoughts of getting home and all the day-to-day tasks ahead.

Lying together in the "spoons position" is a tender way to enjoy those gentle moments after lovemaking.

LOVE-PLAY

"If the lovers spend time playing with and caressing each other both at the beginning and at the end of their loving, then their ecstasy and confidence increase. Love-play enhances pleasure."

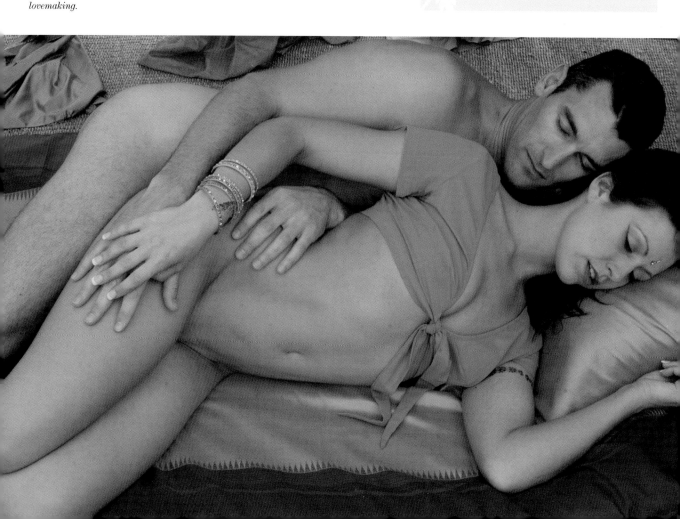

"When a woman is tired, she should place her forehead on that of her lover and should take rest, without disturbing the union of their sex organs. When she has rested herself, the man should turn around and begin to make love with her again."

A CIRCLE OF PLEASURE

With Kama Sutra-style slow loving, there is not necessarily a "final destination" of orgasm. By holding back from climax and staying on an erotically charged plateau of pleasure, lovemaking becomes one continuous movement from foreplay, intercourse, and afterplay flowing into each other in a delicious circle. As Vatsyayana suggests, you may decide to rest with your embers still burning, then continue to play.

STAY IN THE MOMENT

As Vatsyayana suggests, caressing, stroking, and kissing are just as valuable after lovemaking as before. Soft words, appreciating your lover, and sharing thoughts and feelings come naturally in this intimate time—let them flow.

Afterplay also continues long after you've returned from your outdoor adventure and are back in your everyday lives with all the pressures of work and family. A fulfilling and passionate sex life lays firm foundations for closeness throughout your relationship and the bond of intimacy created by shared sexual bliss nourishes the connection with your lover afterward, even when you are apart.

GROUNDING ENERGY

Lovemaking generates huge amounts of powerful energy. If you've ever felt "spaced-out" and light-headed after sex, re-establishing your connection with earth through grounding your energy will allow you to gently re-emerge into the world from the soft space you have been in without losing the blissful sensation.

You might ask your lover to massage your feet gently and hold them enfolded in their hands for a few moments. Other good "earthing" activities to share after sex include eating a little light food and some simple stretches: rise up on your toes, from a standing position, then lower your heels to the ground (bending your knees), feeling yourself push against gravity, and then sinking into it. If there is a stream or pool nearby, why not splash about in it? If you reached your location on foot, you may find that the hike back is itself grounding.

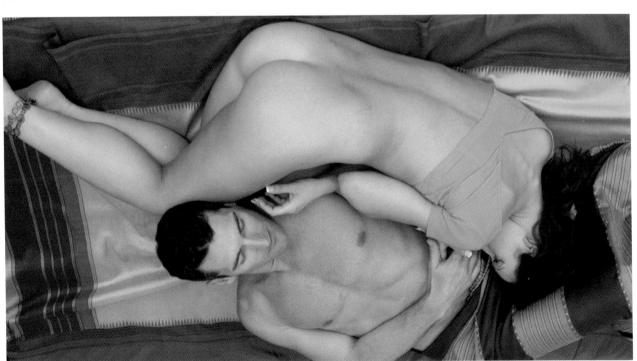

index

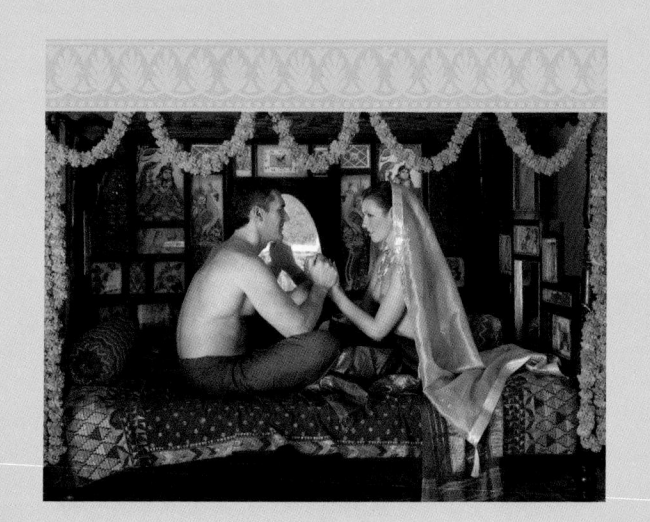

Author's dedication
For Ben, with love